STEWART BRO(

FATTY LIVER
DIET COOKBOOK:

The Ultimate Guide for Managing Liver Health with Over 100 Easy and Healthy Recipes for Beginners, and a 30-Day Fatty Liver Diet Plan to Detox and Cleanse Your Liver

Copyright © 2024

All rights reserved. No part of this publication may be reproduced, distributed, or transmitted in any form or by any means, including photocopying, recording, or other electronic or mechanical methods, without the prior written permission of the publisher, except in the case of brief quotations embodied in critical reviews and certain other noncommercial uses permitted by copyright law. For permission requests, write to the publisher.

The information in this book is provided "as is," without warranty of any kind, express or implied, including but not limited to warranties of merchantability, fitness for a particular purpose, or non-infringement. The content within this book is for informational purposes only and is not intended as medical advice. Consult a healthcare professional before making any changes to your diet or nutrition plan.

The recipes in this cookbook are designed for individuals following a fatty liver diet. However, individual dietary needs may vary. Readers are encouraged to tailor the recipes to their own needs under the guidance of a healthcare professional.

First Edition

This book is a work of authorship and has been written with the intention to provide valuable information to those interested in fatty liver diet cooking. Any resemblances to other works are entirely coincidental.

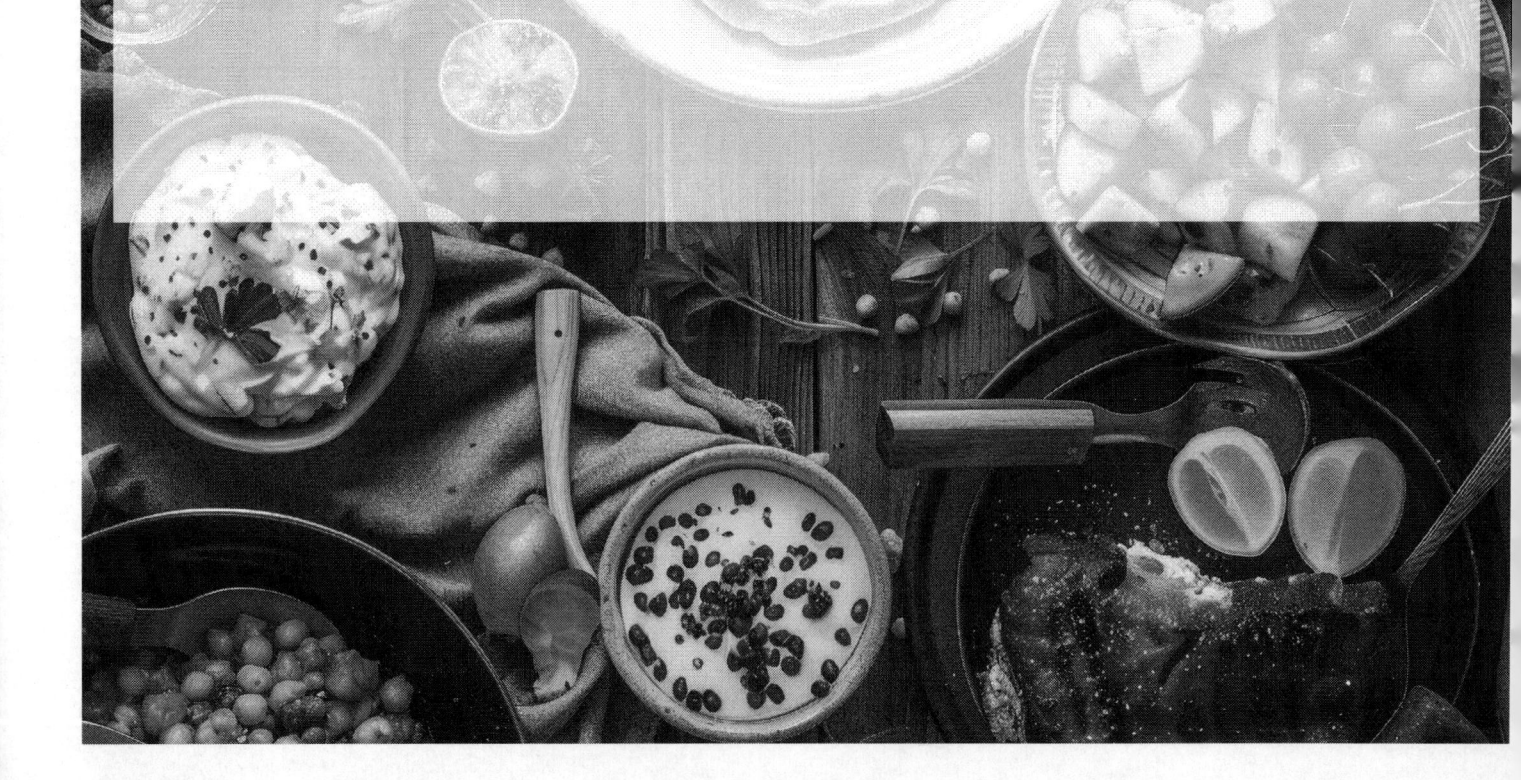

TABLE OF CONTENTS

Introduction: The Journey to a Healthier Liver 7

Chapter 1: Understanding Fatty Liver Disease 10
- What is Fatty Liver Disease? 10
- Types and Causes of Fatty Liver Disease 13
- Symptoms, Diagnosis, and When to Seek Help 15
- Latest Research and Insights into Treatment and Management 17

Chapter 2: Transforming Your Lifestyle for Liver Health 20
- The Role of Lifestyle in Managing Fatty Liver Disease 20
- Holistic Dietary Guidelines for Liver Health 21
- Essential Tips for Meal Planning and Effective Shopping Lists 26
- Kitchen Prep Essentials: Tools and Techniques for Liver-Friendly Cooking 30

Chapter 3: Nourishing Breakfasts to Start Your Day Right 33
- Cottage Cheese Pancakes with Blueberries 34
- Smoked Salmon and Avocado Toast 34
- Easy-to-Follow, Nutritious Breakfast Recipes 34
- Vegan Tofu Scramble with Spinach and Tomatoes 35
- Pear and Walnut Oatmeal 35
- Spiced Pumpkin Porridge 36
- Vegetable Hash with Poached Egg 37
- Walnut and Pear Oat Bake 37
- Salmon and Avocado Toast 38
- Quinoa and Apple Breakfast Bowl 38
- Grilled Chicken and Avocado Wrap 39
- Almond Butter and Banana Oatmeal 39
- Mixed Berry Whole Grain Porridge 40
- Spinach and Egg White Omelette 40
- Mango and Coconut Chia Pudding 41
- Beetroot and Carrot Juice Cleanse 41
- Special Section: Quick Breakfasts for Busy Mornings 41
- Broccoli and Feta Cheese Scramble 42
- Green Tea Yogurt Parfait 42
- Chia Seed and Raspberry Pudding 43
- Whole Wheat Pancakes with Fresh Fruit 43

Chapter 4: Lunches to Love 44
- Quinoa Tabbouleh with Chickpeas 45
- Delicious and Healthy Lunch Recipes 45
- Hearty Minestrone Soup with Whole Wheat Pasta 46
- Grilled Haddock with Olive Tapenade 46
- Carrot and Ginger Purée Soup 47
- Spiced Lentil Stew with Coconut Milk 47
- Tuna and White Bean Salad 48
- Garlic Roasted Trout with Brussels Sprouts 49
- Vegan Buddha Bowl with Spiced Chickpeas 49
- Roasted Vegetable and Farro Bowl 50

Spinach and Mushroom Polenta Stacks 50
Butternut Squash and Chickpea Curry 51
Turmeric Grilled Chicken and Quinoa Salad 51
Asparagus and Shrimp with Quinoa 52
Balsamic Grilled Zucchini with Parmesan 52
Special Section: Lunches on the Go .. 52
Eggplant Rollatini with Spinach and Ricotta 53
Lemon Garlic Tilapia with Steamed Kale 53
Pesto Chicken and Veggie Wrap 54

Chapter 5: Delightful Dinners 55

Pumpkin and Black Bean Casserole .. 56
Creamy Broccoli and Spinach Soup ... 56
Sautéed Brussels Sprouts with Crispy Tofu 57
Stuffed Portobello Mushrooms with Spinach and Pine Nuts 57
Vegetable and Tofu Pad Thai 58
Citrus Roasted Turkey Breast 59
Roasted Cauliflower and Chickpea Tacos 59
Stir-Fried Kale and Quinoa 60
Blackened Catfish with Collard Greens 60
Cod in Parsley Cream Sauce 61
Roasted Beet and Feta Salad 61
Grilled Swordfish with Mediterranean Salad 62
Butternut Squash and Sage Risotto .. 63
Moroccan Spiced Fish with Couscous 64
Baked Hake with Sweet Potato Wedges 64
Spaghetti Squash Pad Thai 65
Spicy Tofu and Bok Choy Stir-Fry 66
Grilled Halibut with Citrus Salsa 66
Miso-Glazed Cod with Bok Choy 67
Roasted Brussels Sprouts and Pomegranate Salad 67
Seared Scallops with Quinoa and Apple Salad 68
Herb Roasted Chicken with Root Vegetables 68
Pumpkin Curry with Brown Rice 69
Vegan Mushroom and Lentil Bolognese 70
Lemon and Herb Poached Haddock .. 70

Chapter 6: Snacks and Appetizers 71

Air-Fried Spiced Carrot Chips 72
Smoked Salmon and Cream Cheese Cucumber Rolls 72
Cucumber Boats with Spicy Shrimp Salad 73
Roasted Brussels Sprouts with Lemon Dip 73
Ricotta and Berry Stuffed Celery 74
Zucchini and Herb Fritters 74
Baked Cod Fish Sticks with Yogurt Dill
Sauce 75
Pumpkin Hummus with Whole Grain Pita Chips 76
Kale and Apple Chips 76
Tahini and Cocoa Energy Bites 77
Stuffed Cherry Tomatoes with Tuna Salad 77
Minty Pea and Avocado Spread on Whole Grain Toast 78

Roasted Turmeric and Cumin Cauliflower Bites..78
No-Bake Walnut and Date Energy Balls..79
Avocado and Lime Frozen Yogurt.....79

Chapter 7: Soups and Stews..80
Cod and Parsnip Stew 81
Black Bean and Butternut Squash Stew..81
Comforting and Healing Soups and Stews..81
Pumpkin and Chickpea Stew...............82
Turkey and Quinoa Stew 83
Mushroom and Barley Soup.................83
Special Section: Quick & Easy One-Pot Wonders..83
Vegetable and Tempeh Stew...............84
Kale and White Bean Soup 85
Spicy Tomato and Lentil Soup............85
Creamy Avocado and Cucumber Soup..86

Chapter 8: Healthy Meat Dishes..87
Moroccan Spiced Chicken Stew with Apricots...88
Asian-Style Turkey Meatballs with Vegetable Stir Fry 89
Stuffed Peppers with Ground Chicken and Brown Rice...................................89
Slow-Cooked Turkey Chili with Sweet Potatoes 90
Balsamic Glazed Duck Breast with
Pear Chutney.......................................90
Beef and Vegetable Kebabs with Tzatziki..91
Stir-Fried Beef and Broccoli with Tamari Sauce..92
Spiced Chicken Skewers with Yogurt Cucumber Dip..92
Spaghetti Squash and Meatballs with Tomato Basil Sauce..............................93

Chapter 9: Flavorful Fish and Seafood..94
Soy-Ginger Glazed Salmon with Bok Choy 95
Parchment-Baked Halibut with Asparagus...95
Horseradish Encrusted Salmon with Beetroot Salad 96
Lemon-Pepper Cod with Broccoli Puree 97
Maple-Glazed Arctic Char with Braised Leeks 97
Spiced Monkfish with Lentil Dal........98
Steamed Mussels with Garlic and Herbs 99
Lemon and Dill Poached Salmon......99
Grilled Tuna with a Citrus Tomato Salsa 100
Miso Glazed Black Cod with Stir-Fried Greens...100

Chapter 10: Desserts...101
Pumpkin Spice Energy Balls...............102
Pineapple Carpaccio with Fresh Basil...102
Avocado Cocoa Mousse.......................103
Baked Grapefruit with Cinnamon...103
Pear and Ginger Compote 104
Roasted Cinnamon Hazelnuts...........104
Blueberry and Lemon Chia Fresca.105
Raspberry Coconut Chia Pudding ..106

Chilled Mango Soup with Mint 106
Fresh Berry Salad with Mint 107
Date and Nut Truffles 107
Coconut and Lime Rice Pudding 108
Baked Peaches with Crushed Almonds 108
Zucchini and Chocolate Chip Bread (Sugar-Free) 109
Sugar-Free Almond Butter Brownies 110

Chapter 11: Hydrating Drinks and Smoothies 111

Carrot, Orange, and Ginger Immune Booster 112
Cucumber, Celery, and Lime Hydration Drink 112
Raspberry, Lime, and Coconut Water Slushie 113
Green Tea Infusion with Mint and Lemon 113
Pineapple and Fresh Turmeric Digestive Aid 114
Matcha and Spirulina Energy Drink ... 114
Soothing Chamomile and Lavender Tea 115
Mango, Kiwi, and Spinach Smoothie 115
Turmeric and Pineapple Anti-Inflammatory Smoothie 116
Pear and Ginger Soother 117

Chapter 12: Comprehensive 30-day Meal Plan 118

Tips for Meal Prep and Storage 120

Chapter 13: Beyond Diet: A Holistic Approach to Liver Health 122

Exercise Recommendations and Tips for Getting Started 122
Stress Reduction Techniques: Meditation, Yoga, and More 123
Navigating Emotional Eating and Building a Support Network 124

Chapter 14: Navigating Challenges and Maintaining Progress 125

How to Adapt Recipes for Different Dietary Needs (Vegan, Gluten-Free, etc.) 125
Overcoming Common Obstacles in Your Diet and Lifestyle Changes 126
Maintaining Motivation and Celebrating Milestones 127
Get your Bonus! 128

Appendix 129

Glossary of Terms 129
Recommended Apps and Online Resources 131

Index 136

INTRODUCTION: THE JOURNEY TO A HEALTHIER LIVER

Welcome to a transformative approach toward enhancing your liver health and overall well-being. Whether diagnosed with fatty liver disease or aiming to boost liver health through proactive dietary adjustments, this cookbook serves as your guide.

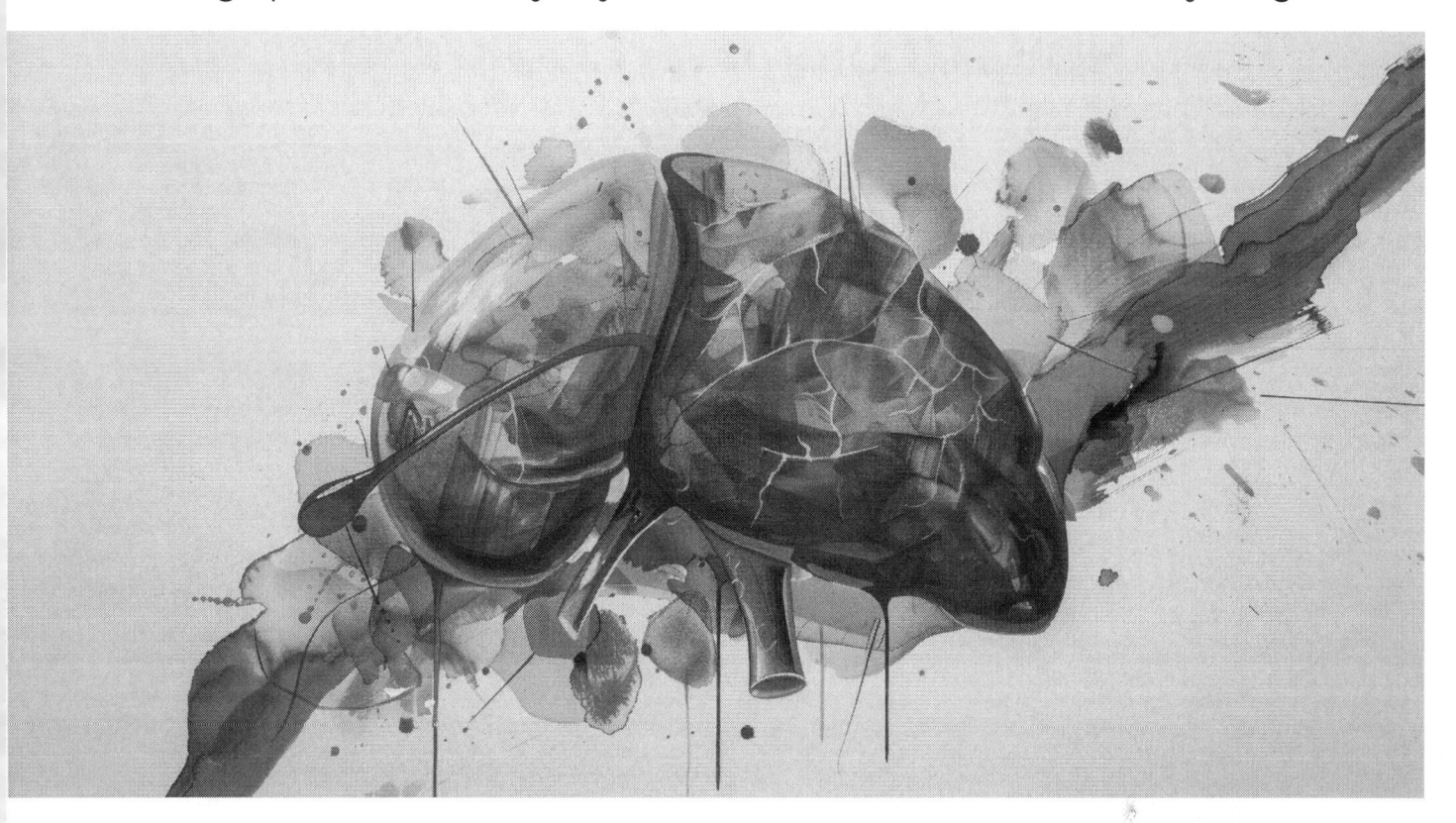

Fatty liver disease is increasingly prevalent, affecting a significant portion of the global population. It is characterized by the excessive accumulation of fats in liver cells, which can lead to more severe health issues if not addressed properly. This book provides practical guidance on combating fatty liver through thoughtful nutrition and beyond. Each section is meticulously crafted to arm you with delicious, liver-friendly recipes and essential knowledge to support your health endeavors.

This book merges the latest scientific insights with actionable advice on lifestyle modifications. From foundational knowledge about fatty liver disease in Chapters 1 and 2 to the adoption of holistic practices for liver health in Chapters 13 and 14, each section builds on the previous to offer a full spectrum of support.

This book is thoughtfully organized to guide you through various aspects of managing fatty liver disease:

- Chapters 1-2 provide essential background on what fatty liver disease entails and the significance of lifestyle in its management.
- Chapters 3-10 form the heart of this cookbook, featuring a range of recipes from breakfasts to desserts, all formulated to be nutritious and supportive of liver health. These chapters also include sections on quick meals.

- Chapter 11 introduces a selection of hydrating drinks and smoothies, while Chapter 12 outlines a structured 30-day meal plan to help you implement the recipes and tips systematically.
- Chapters 13 and 14 broaden the scope beyond diet to include exercise, stress management, emotional eating, and strategies for maintaining motivation — key elements for sustainable lifestyle transformation.

HOW TO USE THIS COOKBOOK

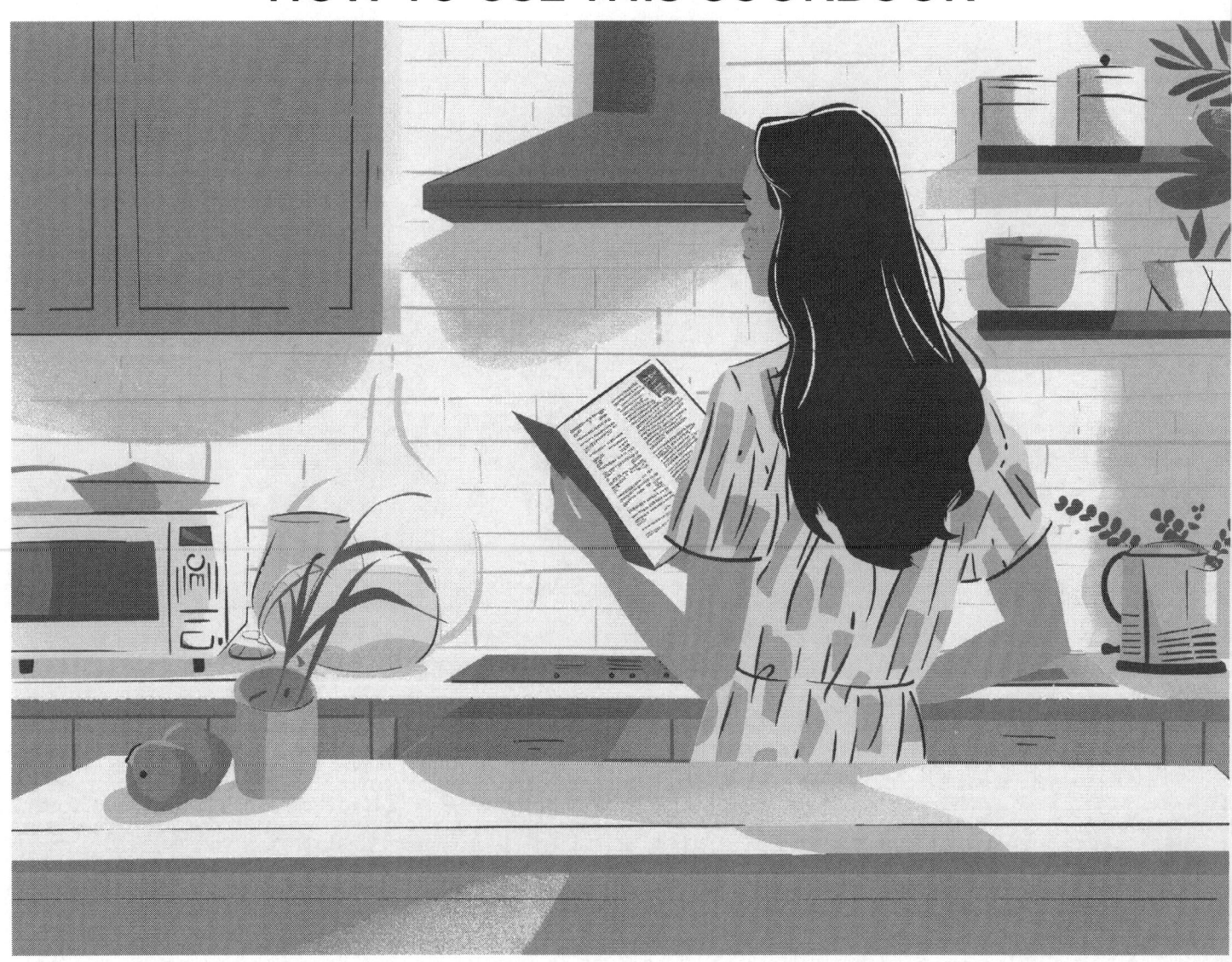

Each recipe in this book comes with detailed instructions and a list of health benefits, helping you understand how each ingredient contributes to liver health. To help you further:

- **Nutritional Profiles:** Detailed information on calorie content, macronutrients, and vitamins present in the recipes helps you track your daily intake and ensures that you're aligning with your health goals.
- **Scalability:** Whether you're cooking for one or for a family, recipes can be easily scaled to accommodate any number of servings, ensuring you can adjust quantities to meet your needs without compromising on taste or nutritional value.

Recipe Tags for Quick Reference

To aid in quick and efficient recipe selection, each recipe is tagged with one or more of the following labels, making it easier for you to find what suits your dietary preferences or needs on any given day:

- **Dietary Preferences:** Tags like Vegan, Vegetarian, Gluten-Free, and Dairy-Free help those with specific dietary restrictions to find suitable recipes quickly.
- **Health Focus:** Tags like Heart-Healthy, Low-Glycemic, High-Protein, and High-Fiber highlight recipes that cater to specific health goals.
- **Nutrient Specific:** Vitamin A, Vitamin C, Vitamin D, and Vitamin E rich tags help those focusing on boosting intake of specific nutrients.

Additional Learning Resources

The Appendix offers a wealth of resources:

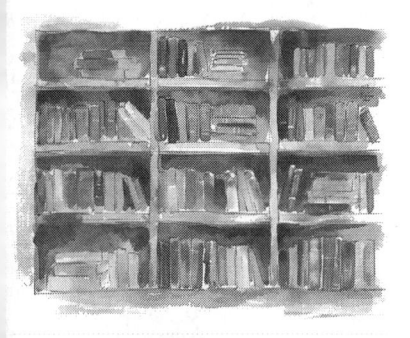

Glossary of Terms: A comprehensive glossary that explains technical terms and ingredients that may be unfamiliar to some readers.

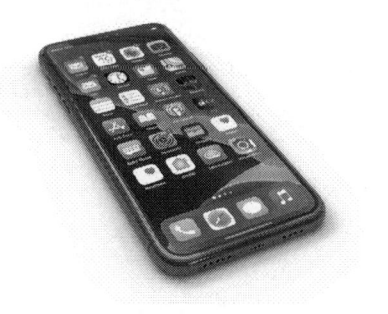

Recommended Apps and Resources: A curated list of apps and websites that provide additional support and tracking capabilities for diet management.

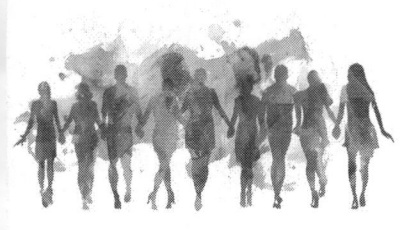

Online Community: Information on how to connect with online forums and groups that can offer support and share experiences related to liver health and healthy eating.

By utilizing this cookbook not just as a collection of recipes but as a holistic guide, you can take meaningful steps towards improving your liver health and enhancing your overall quality of life. This cookbook aims to educate, inspire, and empower you to make informed decisions about your diet and lifestyle.

CHAPTER 1: UNDERSTANDING FATTY LIVER DISEASE

WHAT IS FATTY LIVER DISEASE?

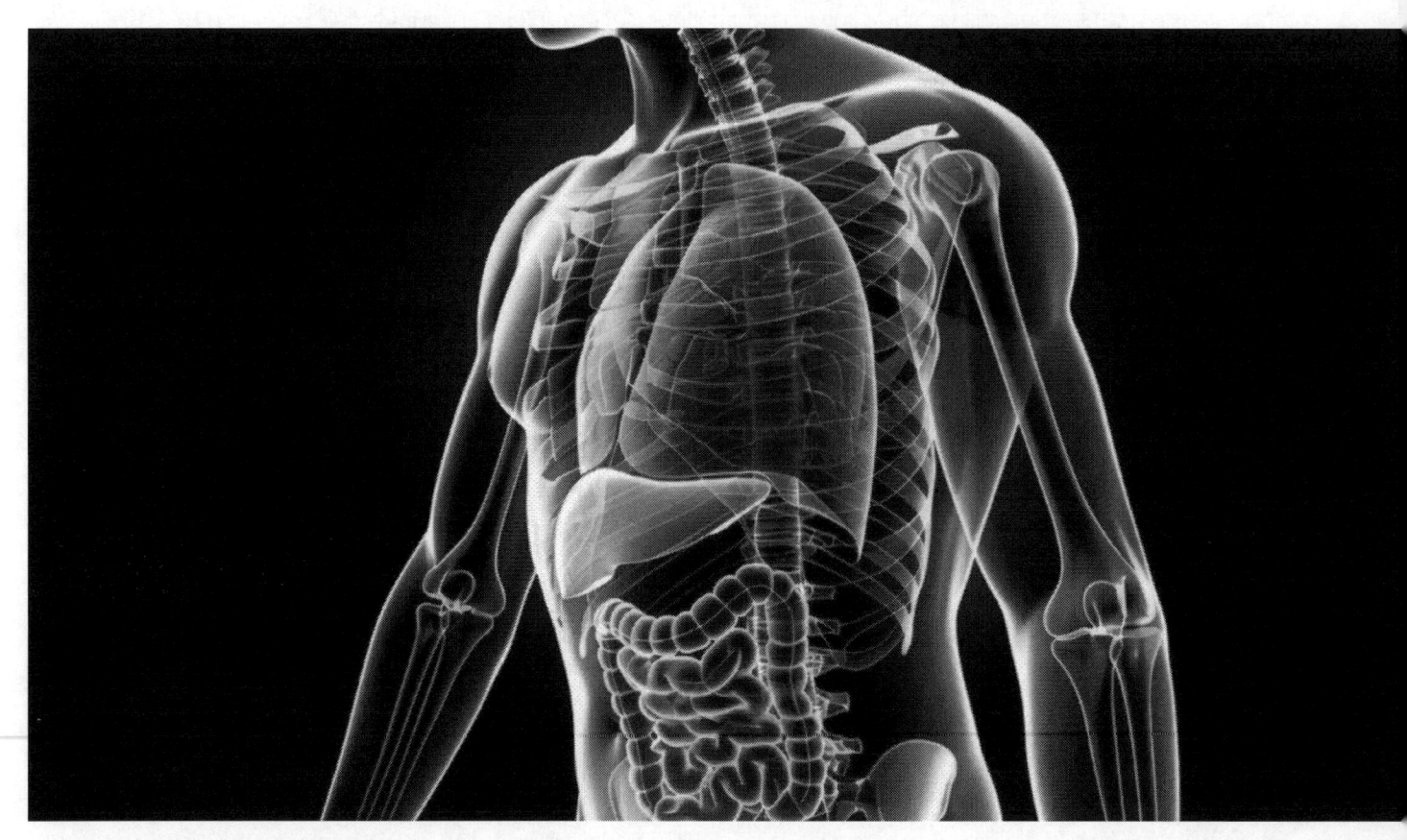

Fatty liver disease, medically known as hepatic steatosis, refers to the accumulation of excess fat in the liver cells. It is a common condition, especially in the United States, where it is closely linked to the rising rates of obesity and type 2 diabetes. Although having small amounts of fat in your liver is normal, excessive fat can cause inflammation and damage, leading to serious health issues, including liver cirrhosis, liver failure, or liver cancer. Understanding this condition is crucial, given its silent progression and significant impact on overall health.

The disease manifests in two main forms: alcoholic fatty liver disease (AFLD) and non-alcoholic fatty liver disease (NAFLD or MASLD). AFLD results from excessive alcohol intake, which directly harms the liver by causing fat to build up in the liver cells. On the other hand, NAFLD, the more common type, occurs in individuals who drink little to no alcohol. Instead, factors like obesity, high cholesterol, high triglycerides, and type 2 diabetes play significant roles in its development. In recent years, NAFLD has become the most common cause of chronic liver disease in the United States, affecting about 25% of the population, including children.

The prevalence of fatty liver disease in America underscores a significant public health challenge. It mirrors the increasing trends of obesity and metabolic syndrome, conditions characterized by high blood pressure, high blood sugar, excess body fat around the waist, and abnormal cholesterol levels. The correlation between fatty liver disease and these metabolic conditions suggests that the American lifestyle, which often involves high-calorie diets and sedentary behavior, is a major contributor to the epidemic.

Despite its high prevalence, fatty liver often remains undiagnosed because it typically does not manifest any symptoms until the liver damage is advanced. When symptoms do appear, they might include fatigue, weakness, weight loss, yellowing of the skin or eyes (jaundice), and discomfort in the upper right abdomen. Due to its silent nature, many individuals are unaware that they have the condition until it is discovered through routine blood tests or check-ups for other medical reasons.

Early detection of fatty liver is essential for effective management and prevention of further complications. Regular check-ups can help catch the disease in its early stages, where interventions such as dietary changes, physical activity, and management of underlying conditions can be most effective. Given the lack of specific medications for treating fatty liver, lifestyle modifications remain the cornerstone of management. These include adopting a healthy diet, engaging in regular physical activity, achieving a healthy weight, and avoiding alcohol consumption.

For Americans, understanding the significance of fatty liver disease and recognizing its risk factors are the first steps toward reversing its course. With its prevalence on the rise, it is more important than ever to be informed about how lifestyle choices can impact liver health. By addressing fatty liver disease proactively through diet and lifestyle changes, individuals can significantly improve their liver function and overall health, reducing the risk of severe liver diseases in the future. This chapter sets the stage for the rest of this cookbook, which will delve into the dietary strategies essential for managing and potentially reversing fatty liver disease.

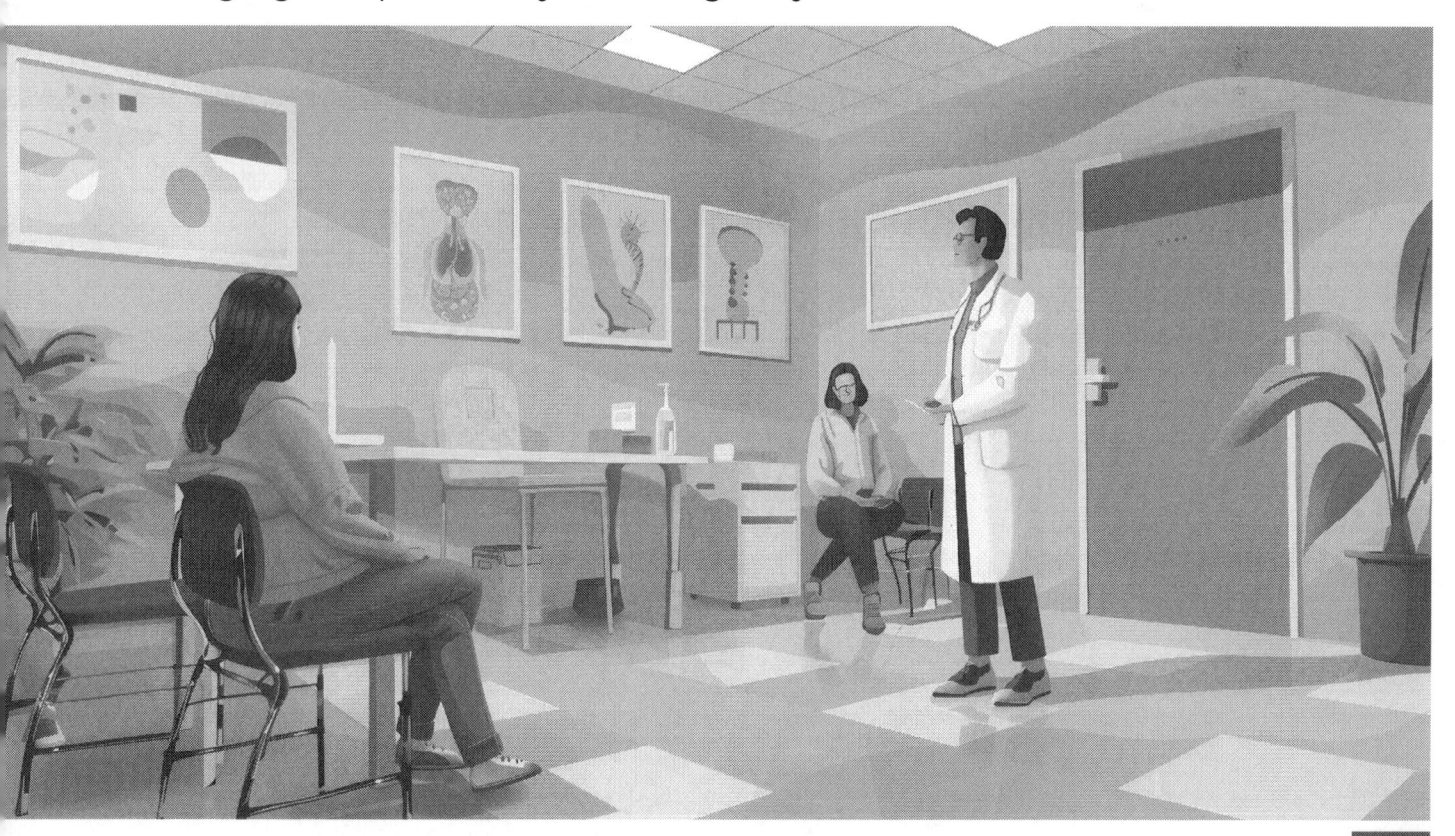

The liver, located just below the diaphragm in the upper right quadrant of the abdomen, is a crucial organ for maintaining overall health. It performs a multitude of essential functions:

Blood Filtration: The liver detoxifies chemicals and metabolizes drugs, filtering blood from the digestive tract before it circulates to the rest of the body. This process helps remove potentially harmful substances consumed or absorbed.

Metabolic Regulation: It regulates the balance of sugar, protein, and fat in the bloodstream. The liver converts excess glucose into glycogen for storage and can also generate glucose when needed, which is vital for energy management.

Bile Production: The liver produces bile, which is essential for fat digestion and the absorption of fat-soluble vitamins (A, D, E, and K). Bile aids in breaking down fats and is critical for proper nutritional absorption.

Blood Clotting: It produces proteins necessary for blood coagulation, playing a key role in healing and preventing excessive bleeding.

Cholesterol Regulation: The liver not only produces cholesterol, crucial for forming cell membranes and certain hormones but also helps remove excess cholesterol from the body, aiding in cardiovascular health.

Maintaining liver health is essential due to its role in these complex functions. A healthy liver ensures efficient performance of these tasks, supporting overall health and preventing diseases. When the liver is damaged, such as with fatty liver disease, its ability to function properly is impaired. This can lead to serious health issues, including the buildup of toxins, poor nutrient digestion and absorption, and metabolic disturbances.

Fatty liver represents a marked deviation from normal liver health, indicated by excessive fat accumulation within liver cells. This condition significantly disrupts the liver's crucial functions and could lead to severe health issues if unchecked. Key points include:

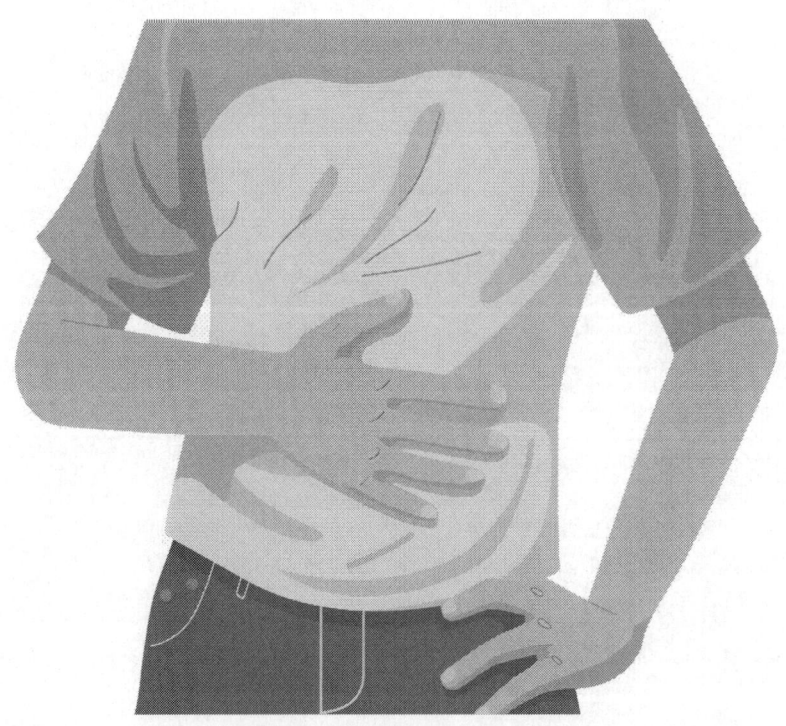

Impact of Disruption: The excess fat can cause cellular dysfunction, inflammatory responses, and fibrosis, potentially progressing to cirrhosis or liver cancer. This disruption affects the body's metabolic balance, influencing cholesterol levels and glucose regulation.

Fatty liver represents a marked deviation from normal liver health, indicated by excessive fat accumulation within liver cells. This condition significantly disrupts the liver's crucial functions and could lead to severe health issues if unchecked. Key points include:

TYPES AND CAUSES OF FATTY LIVER DISEASE

In the exploration of fatty liver disease, it is critical to distinguish between its two main types: alcoholic fatty liver disease (AFLD) and non-alcoholic fatty liver disease (NAFLD). Each type has distinct causes, risk factors, and demographics affected, underscoring the importance of tailored approaches to prevention and treatment.

Alcoholic Fatty Liver Disease (AFLD)

AFLD occurs as a direct result of excessive alcohol consumption. Alcohol metabolism in the liver generates harmful substances that can lead to fat accumulation in liver cells, inflammation, and, eventually, liver damage. The risk of developing AFLD increases with the amount and duration of alcohol consumption. Factors such as genetic predisposition, gender, and underlying health conditions can exacerbate the risk.

Risk Factors:

- Alcohol Consumption: The primary risk factor for AFLD is excessive alcohol intake. The liver processes alcohol, but excessive amounts can overwhelm this process, leading to fat deposition in liver cells.
- Genetic Susceptibility: Genetic factors can influence how the body processes alcohol and how susceptible one is to liver damage. Variations in genes involved in alcohol metabolism can make some individuals more prone to developing AFLD.
- Coexisting Liver Conditions: Individuals with other liver diseases, such as hepatitis C, are more susceptible to harm from alcohol, increasing AFLD risk.

Demographics: Generally, men are more prone to AFLD due to higher rates of alcohol consumption. However, women may be more susceptible to liver damage from alcohol at lower levels of consumption.

Lifestyle and Dietary Contributions:

- Nutritional Deficiencies: Heavy drinkers often have poor dietary habits, leading to deficiencies in nutrients crucial for liver health, such as vitamins A and E, which protect against liver damage.
- Caloric Intake: Excessive alcohol consumption contributes to high caloric intake but poor nutritional value, compounding liver stress and fat accumulation.

Non-Alcoholic Fatty Liver Disease (NAFLD or MASLD)

NAFLD, on the other hand, occurs in individuals who consume little to no alcohol. This type of fatty liver disease is primarily associated with metabolic syndrome, which includes conditions such as obesity, insulin resistance, type 2 diabetes, and dyslipidemia. NAFLD is a reflection of broader lifestyle and health issues prevalent in modern society, particularly in the United States.

Risk Factors:

- Obesity: Especially central obesity, where fat accumulates around the abdomen, significantly increases the risk of NAFLD by promoting insulin resistance and inflammation.
- Type 2 Diabetes: High blood sugar levels can damage tissues, including the liver, making NAFLD more likely.
- Dyslipidemia: High levels of triglycerides and low levels of HDL cholesterol in the blood contribute to fat accumulation in the liver.
- Insulin Resistance: A key component of metabolic syndrome, insulin resistance disrupts normal metabolism and increases fat storage in the liver.
- Genetics: Certain genes affect fat distribution, insulin sensitivity, and the likelihood of inflammation, thereby influencing NAFLD risk.

Demographics: NAFLD is increasingly seen in all age groups but is most common in people in their 40s and 50s due to the accumulation of lifestyle impacts over time. It affects both genders, although slightly more common in men than in women. Ethnicity also plays a role, with Hispanic Americans showing higher prevalence rates, possibly due to higher obesity rates and a genetic predisposition to insulin resistance.

Lifestyle and Dietary Contributions:

- Diet: High intake of refined sugars (especially fructose), saturated fats, and trans fats are linked to increased liver fat and NAFLD. Conversely, a diet rich in whole grains, fruits, vegetables, and healthy fats can help prevent its development.
- Physical Inactivity: Sedentary behavior is associated with higher risk factors for metabolic syndrome, including NAFLD.
- Sleep Patterns: Poor sleep quality and duration can exacerbate metabolic disorders, including obesity and insulin resistance, which in turn can lead to NAFLD.

Shared Risk Factors and Lifestyle Contributions Across AFLD and NAFLD:

- Ethnicity and Demographics: Certain ethnicities, like Hispanic people, have higher rates of metabolic syndrome, contributing to higher NAFLD rates. Conversely, demographic factors such as age and gender also influence the prevalence and progression of both AFLD and NAFLD.
- Socioeconomic Status: Lower socioeconomic status can limit access to healthy food choices and opportunities for physical activity, increasing risk factors associated with both types of fatty liver disease.

The clear differentiation between AFLD and NAFLD not only helps in understanding the specific challenges faced by individuals but also in crafting public health policies and personal health strategies to address these conditions effectively.

SYMPTOMS, DIAGNOSIS, AND WHEN TO SEEK HELP

Symptoms of Fatty Liver Disease

Fatty liver disease often begins silently, with many individuals experiencing no noticeable symptoms during the initial stages of the condition. This asymptomatic nature can make early detection challenging without regular medical screening, particularly in individuals who are at high risk due to underlying health issues like obesity or diabetes.

As the disease progresses to more advanced stages, such as steatohepatitis or fibrosis, symptoms may become more apparent and troublesome. Common symptoms of fatty liver disease include:

Fatigue and Weakness: This is one of the most frequently reported symptoms, where individuals feel a general sense of tiredness that is not relieved by rest. This fatigue can be debilitating and affect daily activities.

Discomfort in the Upper Right Abdomen: Some people may experience dull or aching pain in the upper right area of the abdomen, where the liver is located. This discomfort can sometimes extend to the back or shoulder due to the liver's enlargement or inflammation.

Weight Loss: Unexpected weight loss that occurs without changes in diet or exercise habits can be a sign of advanced fatty liver disease. This symptom often accompanies a loss of appetite.

Jaundice: As liver function worsens, jaundice can develop, which is characterized by a yellowing of the skin and the whites of the eyes. This occurs due to the liver's inability to process bilirubin, a byproduct of old red blood cells.

Swelling: Fluid retention in the abdomen (ascites) and swelling in the legs (edema) can occur as a result of decreased protein production by the liver, which is necessary for maintaining blood pressure and fluid balance within the vessels.

Itchy Skin: Accumulation of bile salts under the skin may cause persistent itching.

Mental Confusion: In severe cases, a buildup of toxins in the bloodstream that are normally cleared by the liver can affect brain function, leading to confusion or difficulty concentrating, known as hepatic encephalopathy.

These symptoms, especially when they appear together, indicate that the liver disease may be advancing and necessitate prompt medical evaluation. Early detection through awareness of symptoms, combined with regular health check-ups, is crucial for managing fatty liver disease effectively and preventing its progression to more serious liver damage.

Diagnostic Process for Fatty Liver Disease

Diagnosing fatty liver disease involves a comprehensive approach that incorporates a combination of physical examinations, laboratory tests, and imaging techniques. Each step is designed to evaluate liver health, confirm the presence of fat accumulation, and assess any resulting damage or inflammation. Here's a detailed look at each component of the diagnostic process:

Physical Exam: During a physical examination, a healthcare provider will look for physical signs of liver disease, such as an enlarged liver or spleen, which can be felt upon palpation of the abdomen. The doctor may also check for other physical indicators, such as jaundice or signs of excess fluid in the abdomen.

Blood Tests: These are critical in the initial screening for fatty liver disease. Liver function tests measure levels of enzymes such as alanine aminotransferase (ALT) and aspartate aminotransferase (AST), which are elevated when liver damage is present. Other tests might include checking for elevated levels of bilirubin and decreased levels of proteins like albumin, which can indicate liver dysfunction. Additionally, blood tests can assess lipid profiles and glucose levels to identify associated conditions like dyslipidemia and diabetes.

Imaging Studies: Imaging techniques play a crucial role in diagnosing fatty liver disease by visually confirming the presence of fat in the liver.

- Ultrasound: This is often the first imaging test used because it's non-invasive, widely available, and cost-effective. An ultrasound can detect increased liver echogenicity, suggesting fat deposition.
- Computed Tomography (CT) Scan: While not as sensitive as other methods for detecting liver fat, a CT scan can help assess liver size and rule out other abnormalities.
- Magnetic Resonance Imaging (MRI): This is more sensitive than ultrasound and can be used to quantify the amount of fat in the liver. However, it's more expensive and less widely available.

Liver Biopsy: Considered the gold standard for diagnosing fatty liver disease, a liver biopsy involves removing a small sample of liver tissue with a needle. The sample is then examined under a microscope to determine the extent of fat accumulation, inflammation, and fibrosis. While invasive, a biopsy is the most definitive way to assess liver health and the stage of any disease.

Transient Elastography (FibroScan): This non-invasive test measures liver stiffness, which correlates with fibrosis. It's increasingly used to assess the severity of liver scarring without the need for a biopsy.

Advanced Blood Tests: Some newer blood tests can measure biomarkers related to liver fibrosis and inflammation, offering additional non-invasive options for assessing liver health.

The combination of these diagnostic tools allows for a comprehensive evaluation of the liver's condition. It's essential for individuals at risk of fatty liver disease to undergo these diagnostic tests if they exhibit symptoms or if routine screenings suggest liver abnormalities. Early diagnosis is crucial for effective management and prevention of progressive liver damage.

When to Seek Medical Advice

Early detection of fatty liver disease is critical for preventing serious health complications. Guidance on when to seek medical advice includes:

Risk Factor Awareness: Individuals with risk factors such as obesity, diabetes, high cholesterol, or a history of heavy alcohol use should discuss liver health with their healthcare provider.

Regular Check-Ups: Routine health evaluations can help catch liver abnormalities early, even before symptoms appear. Regular blood tests can monitor liver enzyme levels, which might indicate the need for further investigation.

Symptom Observation: Anyone experiencing symptoms associated with liver disease, such as unexplained fatigue, abdominal discomfort, or jaundice, should consult their doctor promptly.

Lifestyle Changes: Those diagnosed with or at risk for fatty liver disease should regularly consult their healthcare provider to monitor their condition and the effectiveness of lifestyle modifications.

Proactive medical consultation and regular health monitoring play essential roles in managing fatty liver disease, enabling early intervention and preventing progression to more severe liver conditions.

LATEST RESEARCH AND INSIGHTS INTO TREATMENT AND MANAGEMENT

The latest research and advancements in the treatment and management of fatty liver disease, particularly non-alcoholic steatohepatitis (NASH), have been marked by significant milestones, including the FDA approval of the first drug specifically designed to treat this condition. This development represents a critical step forward in the medical community's ability to combat a disease that has long lacked a dedicated therapy.

Differences Between NAFLD and NASH

NAFLD is a broader term that includes any form of liver fat accumulation without significant alcohol consumption. In contrast, NASH specifically refers to the presence of liver inflammation and damage in addition to fat. Not everyone with NAFLD progresses to NASH, but NASH represents a serious progression that increases the risk of further complications like liver fibrosis, cirrhosis, and even liver cancer.

The FDA's recent approval of Rezdiffra (Resmetirom) marks a breakthrough in the treatment of NASH. Rezdiffra works by targeting and activating the thyroid hormone receptor selectively within the liver. This activation is designed to reduce liver fat, inflammation, and fibrosis without eliciting the common side effects associated with thyroid hormone therapy, such as impacts on heart rate and bone health. This treatment offers hope not just for managing NASH but potentially reversing its effects. The approval was based on extensive clinical trials demonstrating the drug's efficacy in reducing liver fat and improving liver health markers.

In the evolving landscape of liver disease terminology, there has been a significant shift in naming conventions to better reflect the underlying causes and characteristics of these conditions. The terms non-alcoholic fatty liver disease (NAFLD) and non-alcoholic steatohepatitis (NASH) have been updated to metabolic dysfunction-associated steatotic liver disease (MASLD) and metabolic dysfunction-associated steatohepatitis (MASH), respectively. This change aims to more accurately describe these diseases as part of a broader spectrum of metabolic dysfunction rather than merely focusing on the absence of alcohol consumption.

Treatment Options

Treatment strategies for **NAFLD** primarily focus on managing the underlying metabolic conditions and lifestyle factors contributing to liver fat accumulation:

- Lifestyle Modifications: This is the first-line treatment for NAFLD, involving dietary changes to reduce weight, increase physical activity, and improve diet quality, particularly reducing intake of saturated fats and sugars.
- Medical Treatments: While there are no FDA-approved drugs specifically for NAFLD (aside from the newly approved Rezdiffra for NASH), treatments may involve managing associated conditions such as diabetes, obesity, and hyperlipidemia with relevant medications.

For **NASH**, the recent approval of Rezdiffra (Resmetirom) marks a significant advancement:

- Rezdiffra (Resmetirom): This is the first drug specifically approved for NASH and works by targeting and activating the thyroid hormone receptor selectively within the liver, helping reduce liver fat, inflammation, and fibrosis.

Alcoholic fatty liver disease (**AFLD**), on the other hand, results from excessive alcohol intake and has different treatment protocols:

- Abstinence from Alcohol: Complete cessation of alcohol intake is the most effective treatment for reversing the effects of AFLD.
- Nutritional Support and Lifestyle Changes: Addressing nutritional deficiencies and maintaining a healthy lifestyle are crucial for liver recovery in AFLD patients

The Role of Diet and Lifestyle Modifications

Despite the advancement in drug treatments, diet, and lifestyle modifications remain foundational in managing and potentially reversing fatty liver disease. These include:

- Diet: Adhering to a healthy diet, such as the Mediterranean diet, which is low in saturated and trans fats and high in fiber, helps manage body weight and reduces liver fat.
- Physical Activity: Regular exercise helps reduce liver fat and improve liver function.
- Weight Management: Maintaining a healthy weight through a balanced diet and regular exercise is crucial; even a modest weight loss of 5-10% can significantly improve liver health.

As we conclude this chapter on understanding fatty liver disease, it is crucial to recognize the dynamic nature of medical research and its ongoing impact on the management and treatment of liver conditions such as NAFLD and NASH. The field of medicine is continually evolving, with new discoveries and advancements that enhance our understanding and improve our approaches to these complex diseases.

It is essential for individuals facing liver health challenges to stay informed about the latest developments and consult healthcare professionals to discuss their specific conditions and treatment options. This is especially important as new treatments like Rezdiffra become available and as our understanding of the genetic, lifestyle, and environmental factors contributing to liver disease deepens. Engaging with a medical professional ensures that treatment plans are based on the most current knowledge and tailored to individual needs.

Further research into the studies mentioned and beyond is highly recommended for those interested in a deeper understanding of fatty liver disease. This can provide invaluable insights into the nuances of treatment options and the latest scientific advancements.

This book, focusing specifically on diet, weight management, and physical activity, highlights aspects of liver health management that are universally necessary. Regardless of the type of liver disease, these elements form the cornerstone of liver health and general well-being. By maintaining a healthy diet, managing weight, and staying active, individuals can significantly impact their liver condition and overall health, often preventing the progression of diseases such as NAFLD and NASH.

In essence, while this chapter provides a foundation of knowledge, continuous learning, and consultation with healthcare providers are key to effectively managing liver health. By staying engaged with the latest medical research and actively participating in your healthcare decisions, you can better navigate the challenges of liver disease and lead a healthier life.

CHAPTER 2: TRANSFORMING YOUR LIFESTYLE FOR LIVER HEALTH

THE ROLE OF LIFESTYLE IN MANAGING FATTY LIVER DISEASE

Fatty liver disease, particularly non-alcoholic fatty liver disease (NAFLD) and its more severe form, non-alcoholic steatohepatitis (NASH), has become increasingly prevalent worldwide, largely due to lifestyle factors associated with modern living. The good news is that lifestyle modifications can significantly impact the management and progression of these conditions. This section will explore how lifestyle choices influence liver health, the effectiveness of lifestyle changes in managing fatty liver disease, and the scientific evidence supporting these approaches.

Impact of Lifestyle Choices on Liver Health

The liver plays a crucial role in metabolizing nutrients, detoxifying harmful substances, and regulating metabolism. Lifestyle choices directly impact liver function and can either support liver health or contribute to liver damage. Poor dietary choices, lack of physical activity, excessive alcohol consumption, and tobacco use are known risk factors that contribute to the accumulation of fat in the liver, leading to NAFLD.

Over time, consistent dietary excesses, especially high intakes of sugars (fructose) and saturated fats, can lead to an increased accumulation of fat in liver cells. This not only burdens the liver's ability to function normally but also predisposes it to inflammation, which can progress to more severe liver damage if unchecked. Similarly, physical inactivity can exacerbate the risk of obesity and insulin resistance, further increasing the risk of developing fatty liver disease.

Modifications in Diet, Physical Activity, and Lifestyle Factors

Modifying one's diet and increasing physical activity are primary steps in managing or preventing fatty liver disease. A liver-friendly diet typically includes:

- **Reduced intake of saturated fats and sugars:** Reducing foods high in saturated fats and sugars, especially fructose, which is commonly found in sweetened beverages and snacks, can decrease liver fat accumulation.

- **Increased intake of fiber and healthy fats:** Diets rich in vegetables, fruits, whole grains, and healthy fats, such as those found in fish, nuts, and olive oil, can help improve liver health. These foods help balance blood sugar levels and reduce liver fat.

- **Moderate, regular physical activity:** Exercise helps to burn triglycerides for fuel and can reduce liver fat. Recommendations typically include at least 150 minutes of moderate-intensity exercise per week, such as brisk walking, cycling, or swimming.

Lifestyle modifications, including achieving a healthy weight, can also significantly impact liver health. Even a modest weight loss of 5% to 10% of body weight is associated with a reduction in liver fat and improvements in various biomarkers of liver function.

Evidence from Recent Studies

Recent studies provide compelling evidence supporting the role of lifestyle changes in improving liver health among patients with fatty liver disease. Research has shown that dietary modifications, along with regular physical activity, not only reduce liver fat but also improve liver enzyme levels and liver fibrosis.

- **Dietary impacts:** Studies have demonstrated that diets low in carbohydrates, particularly sugars, and high in fiber can lead to significant reductions in liver fat content. The Mediterranean diet, for instance, has been extensively studied and shown to be effective in reducing liver fat, improving insulin sensitivity, and even reversing NAFLD in some cases.
- **Physical activity:** Regular physical activity is known to improve antioxidant levels, reduce oxidative stress, and decrease liver fat. Exercise protocols ranging from resistance training to aerobic exercises have all been shown to be beneficial in reducing liver fat independent of weight loss.
- **Holistic lifestyle changes:** Comprehensive lifestyle prog that incorporate both dietary changes and regular physical activity are particularly effective. Such prog not only improve liver enzyme profiles and reduce liver fat but also enhance overall metabolic health, thereby tackling the root causes of fatty liver disease.

HOLISTIC DIETARY GUIDELINES FOR LIVER HEALTH

Adopting a holistic approach to nutrition is crucial for maintaining liver health. This section will provide a comprehensive overview of dietary recommendations aimed at supporting optimal liver function, focusing on a balanced intake of macronutrients and micronutrients, highlighting beneficial foods, and discussing foods that should be limited or avoided.

Balanced Intake of Macronutrients and Micronutrients

The liver plays a pivotal role in metabolizing nutrients; therefore, a balanced diet that supports liver health should include an appropriate mix of macronutrients—carbohydrates, proteins, and fats—alongside essential micronutrients.

- **Carbohydrates:** Opt for complex carbohydrates that are high in fiber, such as whole grains, legumes, and vegetables. Fiber aids digestion and helps regulate blood sugar levels, preventing the liver from being overloaded with insulin and glucose.
- **Proteins:** Adequate protein intake is vital for liver repair and the prevention of muscle wasting. Sources of lean protein such as chicken, fish, tofu, and legumes are recommended. These proteins provide essential amino acids without excessive fats.

- **Fats:** Healthy fats, particularly those rich in omega-3 fatty acids like those found in fish, nuts, and seeds, can help reduce liver fat levels and inflammation. It is crucial to moderate the intake of saturated fats and entirely avoid trans fats.

Micronutrients play specific roles in liver health:

- Vitamins such as **Vitamin E** and **Vitamin D** have been shown to improve liver function in individuals with fatty liver disease. Vitamin E acts as an antioxidant, while Vitamin D has anti-inflammatory effects.
- Minerals like **zinc** and **selenium** are also essential, as they help protect the liver from damage due to their antioxidant properties.

Foods to Support Liver Function

Certain foods are particularly beneficial for liver health:

Leafy Greens

Leafy green vegetables such as spinach, kale, and swiss chard are powerhouse foods for liver health. These vegetables are high in chlorophyll, which naturally assists the liver in clearing toxins from the bloodstream. Leafy greens also offer a protective effect due to their high levels of antioxidants and vitamins that help reduce inflammation and oxidative stress. The fiber content in these greens aids in digestion and helps maintain steady blood sugar levels, thus reducing the liver's workload.

Cruciferous Vegetables

Broccoli, Brussels sprouts, and cauliflower are examples of cruciferous vegetables that are particularly beneficial for the liver. These vegetables are rich in glucosinolates, compounds that help the liver produce enzymes used in the detoxification process. These enzymes aid in flushing out carcinogens and other toxins from the body, enhancing liver health. Regular consumption of cruciferous vegetables has been linked to a lower risk of liver cancer.

Fatty Fish

Fatty fish like salmon, mackerel, and sardines are rich in omega-3 fatty acids, which are known to reduce inflammation and have been found to help lower liver fat levels and decrease inflammation in individuals with fatty liver disease. Omega-3 fatty acids also help maintain enzyme levels and improve insulin sensitivity, which are crucial for individuals with fatty liver disease.

Nuts

Nuts, especially walnuts, are high in omega-3 fatty acids and antioxidants, which support liver health by preventing the accumulation of fat and maintaining normal enzyme levels in the liver. They also contain the amino acid arginine, which helps detoxify ammonia. Walnuts also boost glutathione and omega-3 fatty acid levels in the liver, aiding its cleansing processes.

Garlic

Garlic is a superfood beneficial for liver health due to its high levels of allicin, a compound known for its antioxidant, antibiotic, and antifungal properties. Garlic helps stimulate the liver to activate enzymes that flush out toxins. It also has a significant impact on reducing body weight and fat content, which can help prevent or alleviate non-alcoholic fatty liver disease.

Turmeric

Turmeric is another liver-friendly spice, largely due to its active ingredient, curcumin, which is known for its potent antioxidant and anti-inflammatory properties. Curcumin helps protect the liver from damage by toxins, promotes the regeneration of damaged liver cells, and enhances bile production, which aids in digestion.

Green Tea

Rich in antioxidants known as catechins, green tea supports overall health and improves liver function. The antioxidant properties of green tea help in reducing oxidative stress and fat deposits in the liver, which are crucial in treating and preventing fatty liver disease.

Incorporating these foods into your diet can significantly contribute to liver health and prevent liver diseases. Regular consumption, combined with an overall healthy lifestyle and diet, provides the best protective measures for maintaining a healthy liver. Each of these foods brings a unique set of nutrients that help cleanse, protect, and regenerate liver cells, underscoring the vital role of diet in liver health.

Foods to Avoid or Minimize

To effectively manage or prevent fatty liver disease and other liver conditions, it is crucial to be aware of certain foods that can exacerbate liver issues. These include items high in saturated fats, sugars, and processed ingredients. Below, we explore why these foods are harmful to liver health and provide guidelines on how to minimize their consumption.

High Saturated Fats and Trans Fats

Foods rich in saturated fats and trans fats can contribute to the buildup of liver fat. Saturated fats are typically found in animal products such as red meat, full-fat dairy products, and certain oils (like palm and coconut oil). These fats can increase liver fat, which is especially problematic in individuals with existing liver conditions.

Trans fats are even more detrimental. Often present in fried foods, baked goods, and processed snacks, trans fats are created by adding hydrogen to vegetable oil (a process known as hydrogenation) to increase the shelf life of foods. Consumption of trans fats has been linked to increased inflammation and a higher risk of liver fibrosis, which involves thickening and scarring of liver tissue.

Sugars, Especially Fructose

Excessive intake of sugars, particularly fructose, plays a significant role in the development of fatty liver disease. Fructose is metabolized directly by the liver and, in large amounts, can lead to increased fat buildup within liver cells. Foods high in added sugars, such as sodas, sweets, and desserts, as well as sweetened beverages, should be consumed sparingly. The American Heart Association suggests limiting added sugars to no more than 36 g (9 teaspoons) per day for men and 25 g (6 teaspoons) for women.

Processed Foods

Processed foods are often high in calories, fats, and sodium but low in nutrients, making them particularly harmful to liver health. These foods typically contain additives and preservatives that can place additional stress on the liver. Examples include fast food, packaged snacks, and convenience meals. Processed foods can also contain high levels of refined carbohydrates, which contribute to liver fat accumulation and insulin resistance.

Alcohol

While alcohol is more directly linked to alcoholic liver disease, even those with non-alcoholic fatty liver disease should consider minimizing alcohol consumption. Alcohol can exacerbate liver inflammation and damage, and reducing intake can significantly benefit liver health.

Practical Tips for Minimizing Harmful Foods:

- **Read Labels:** Become vigilant about reading food labels to avoid high-fat, high-sugar, and high-sodium products.
- **Cook at Home:** Preparing meals at home can help control the quality of ingredients and avoid harmful additives found in many processed foods.
- **Choose Healthier Alternatives:** Opt for fresh or frozen fruits and vegetables instead of canned or processed versions, and select lean cuts of meat or plant-based proteins over fatty meats.

For better understanding, here is a table of foods to avoid and why:

FOOD NAME	WHY YOU SHOULD AVOID IT
Pizza	Often loaded with high-fat cheeses and processed meats, contributing to high saturated fat intake.
Bacon	High in saturated fats and sodium, can increase the risk of liver damage.
Doughnuts	High in trans fats and sugars, leading to fat accumulation in the liver.
Ice Cream	Contains high amounts of sugar and saturated fats, problematic for liver health.
Potato Chips	Fried in unhealthy oils and high in trans fats and sodium.
Margarine	Often made with hydrogenated oils, a source of trans fats.
Fried Chicken	The frying process introduces trans fats, which are harmful to the liver.
Canned Soup	Usually contains large amounts of sodium, which can burden the liver.
White Bread	Made from refined flour and often high in sugar, contributes to insulin resistance and liver fat storage.
Sweetened Beverages	High in fructose, which is processed by the liver and can lead to fatty liver disease.
Fast Food Burgers	Typically high in calories, fats, and sodium, all of which are stressors on liver function.
Pastries and Cakes	Loaded with sugars and fats, which can contribute to liver fat.
French Fries	High in trans fats and refined carbohydrates, leading to increased liver fat.
Full-Fat Cheese	High in saturated fat, which can contribute to liver fat accumulation.
Candy Bars	High sugar content can lead to increased liver fat and inflammation.
Regular Soda	Another major source of fructose, linked to increased liver fat and potential liver damage.
Packaged Snacks	Often contain both high levels of sodium and trans fats.
Fried Snacks	Similar to fried chicken, these are often cooked in unhealthy oils and fats.
Store-Bought Smoothies	Can be deceptive; often laden with sugars and calories that are harmful to liver health.
Energy Drinks	High in sugars and other chemicals that can overload the liver.

Implementing Dietary Changes

Successfully adopting these dietary guidelines requires thoughtful meal planning and a commitment to making healthier food choices consistently. It involves reading labels, preparing meals at home, and being mindful of portion sizes. Over time, these changes can significantly improve liver health and overall wellness.

By focusing on a diet rich in whole foods and balanced in essential nutrients while avoiding harmful fats and sugars, individuals can effectively support and enhance liver function. This approach not only helps in managing liver disease but also contributes to a healthier lifestyle overall, proving beneficial for long-term well-being.

ESSENTIAL TIPS FOR MEAL PLANNING AND EFFECTIVE SHOPPING LISTS

Embarking on a liver-friendly diet requires thoughtful meal planning and careful shopping. This section provides practical advice on how to plan meals that align with the dietary guidelines for liver health, create effective shopping lists, and integrate these habits into your daily routine seamlessly.

Planning Meals for Liver Health

Firstly, it's important to understand what your liver needs to function optimally. A diet beneficial for liver health should include:

- **Low Levels of Saturated Fats:** A high intake of saturated fats is linked to liver disease; opting for lean meats and plant-based proteins can help manage this risk.
- **High Fiber Foods:** Fiber helps control blood sugar levels and assists in digestion, which reduces stress on the liver. Include plenty of fruits, vegetables, and whole grains.
- **Antioxidant-Rich Foods:** Foods high in antioxidants help protect the liver by reducing oxidative stress. Incorporate berries, nuts, and leafy greens into your diet.

Each meal should have a good balance of macronutrients:

- **Proteins:** Choose lean protein sources such as fish, poultry, beans, and legumes. These foods provide essential amino acids without excessive fats.
- **Carbohydrates:** Focus on complex carbohydrates like whole grains and vegetables, which provide energy and essential nutrients without spiking blood sugar levels.
- **Fats:** Include healthy fats from sources like avocados, olive oil, and fatty fish. These fats are essential for nutrient absorption and reducing inflammation.

Plan to eat at regular intervals to maintain steady energy levels and avoid overloading the liver with large meals. Small, frequent meals are often recommended:

- **Breakfast:** Start with a nutrient-rich breakfast to activate your metabolism. Include a good source of protein and fiber to keep you full and energized.
- **Lunch and Dinner:** Keep these meals balanced with a variety of food groups, fo-

cusing on vegetables, proteins, and healthy fats.
- **Snacks:** Choose snacks that are high in fiber and protein to keep you satisfied between meals and prevent sudden hunger pangs.

Diversity in your diet ensures you get a range of nutrients that helps keep your meals interesting and enjoyable:
- **Rotate Your Greens:** Use a variety of leafy greens throughout the week, such as spinach, kale, and romaine.
- **Vary Your Proteins:** Alternate between different proteins to avoid monotony and balance the types of amino acids and other nutrients you consume.
- **Experiment with Whole Grains:** Beyond brown rice and whole wheat, try grains like quinoa, barley, and bulgur.

Creating Effective Shopping Lists

Creating an effective shopping list is key to adhering to a liver-friendly diet. This process ensures that you purchase all the necessary ingredients to make healthy meals throughout the week, minimizing the temptation to indulge in less healthy options. Here's how to optimize your shopping list for liver health, with a special focus on reading labels.

Organize Your List by Meal Components

Start by categorizing your list into sections such as proteins, vegetables, fruits, grains, dairy, and pantry staples. This not only helps streamline your shopping process, ensuring you don't miss any items, but also aids in balancing your cart with a variety of food groups. For example:
- Proteins: List chicken, fish, tofu, and legumes.
- Vegetables and Fruits: Include a variety of colors and types, such as leafy greens, berries, oranges, and beets.
- Whole Grains: Opt for quinoa, whole wheat pasta, and brown rice.
- Healthy Fats: Include items like avocados, olive oil, and nuts.

Focus on Fresh and Whole Foods: Prioritize fresh produce and whole ingredients, as these are typically richer in nutrients and free from unnecessary additives. Fresh foods are foundational to a liver-friendly diet, providing the vitamins, minerals, and other nutrients that support liver health.

Make Use of Technology: Use apps or digital tools that can help in planning and organizing your shopping lists. Many apps allow you to save lists, share them with family members, and even order groceries online, which can save time and help you avoid impulse buys. For more information on useful apps, check out the "Recommended Apps and Online Resources" chapter.

Reading Labels

When purchasing packaged foods, reading labels is crucial to avoid ingredients that may harm liver health. Here are key things to look for:

- **Check for Serving Size:** This will help you understand how much of each nutrient you will be consuming.
- **Limit Added Sugars:** Look out for high levels of sugars, especially added sugars like high-fructose corn syrup, which are harmful to liver health.
- **Avoid Unhealthy Fats:** Steer clear of trans fats and limit saturated fats. These can often be hidden in baked goods, fried foods, and snacks.
- **Watch for Sodium:** Excessive sodium intake can be detrimental to liver health, especially if water retention is a concern.
- **Look for Fiber:** High fiber content is a good sign, especially in bread, cereals, and snacks.

Here's a table listing specific ingredients to avoid on food labels, along with reasons why they are detrimental to liver health:

INGREDIENT	REASON TO AVOID
Trans Fats	Can lead to increased liver fat and inflammation. Often listed as "partially hydrogenated oils."
High Fructose Corn Syrup	Contributes to fat buildup in the liver and can exacerbate liver disease.
Added Sugars	Excessive sugar intake can lead to obesity, insulin resistance, and fatty liver. Look for names like sucrose, glucose, and fructose.
Sodium	High sodium levels can contribute to water retention and high blood pressure, stressing the liver.
Artificial Sweeteners	While not directly harmful to the liver, they can negatively affect gut health and glucose tolerance.
Artificial Preservatives	Chemicals such as nitrates and nitrites can be hard on the liver and other organs.
Artificial Colors	Some synthetic dyes have been linked to health issues, though not always directly to liver damage.
Saturated Fats	High levels can contribute to liver fat accumulation. Commonly found in fatty cuts of meat, full-fat dairy, and certain oils.
Alcohol	Directly toxic to liver cells, alcohol can cause inflammation, fat buildup, and eventually liver fibrosis.

A table highlighting key ingredients to look for on labels, which can help guide your decisions:

INGREDIENT	BENEFIT OR REASON TO CHOOSE
Fiber	Look for high fiber content, especially in bread, cereals, and legumes, as fiber helps with digestion and can regulate blood sugar levels.
Omega-3 Fatty Acids	Beneficial for reducing inflammation. Common in fish oils and flaxseeds. Ideal for heart and liver health.
Unsaturated Fats	Healthier fat choices (monounsaturated and polyunsaturated fats), such as those found in olive oil, nuts, and avocados, support overall heart and liver health.
Whole Grains	Whole grains should be the first ingredient in bread and cereals, indicating a good source of fiber and nutrients.
Low Sodium	Choose products with low sodium content to help maintain healthy blood pressure and reduce liver strain.
No Added Sugars	Avoid products with added sugars like sucrose, glucose, or high-fructose corn syrup, especially important for liver health.
Natural Ingredients	Opt for products with natural and recognizable ingredients over those with artificial additives and preservatives.
Probiotics	Found in some yogurts and fermented foods, probiotics support digestive health, which can indirectly benefit liver function.
Antioxidants	Ingredients like vitamins C and E, selenium, and beta-carotene help protect the body and liver from oxidative stress.

Prepare for Impulse Buys: Even with a well-planned list, impulse buys can happen. Prepare for this by allocating a small part of your list to 'free-choice' items that might not be essential but are still within the healthy range. This can satisfy cravings without compromising the overall quality of your diet.

Review and Adjust: After shopping, review what items you bought that were not on your list and reflect on why. Understanding your shopping habits can help you refine future lists and make more mindful choices.

By following these guidelines, you can create shopping lists that not only adhere to dietary needs but also enhance your overall approach to eating for liver health. Preparing a thoughtful list based on organized categories, focusing on fresh ingredients, using technological aids, and reading labels carefully can transform how you shop and eat, promoting better liver health and general well-being.

KITCHEN PREP ESSENTIALS: TOOLS AND TECHNIQUES FOR LIVER-FRIENDLY COOKING

Creating a liver-friendly kitchen starts with having the right tools and techniques to prepare healthy meals. This part of the chapter will explore essential kitchen tools and appliances, discuss cooking techniques that preserve the nutritional integrity of foods, and provide guidance on portion control and meal balance. These elements are crucial for supporting liver health through diet.

Essential Kitchen Tools and Appliances

- Blenders and Food Processors: Blenders are ideal for making smoothies, which are a fantastic way to consume a variety of fruits, vegetables, and other liver-friendly ingredients like flaxseeds or wheatgerm. Food processors are excellent for preparing homemade dips, salsas, and purees, which can be healthier than store-bought versions that may contain excess sodium and preservatives.
- Grills and Grill Pans: Grilling is a healthy cooking method that adds flavor without the need for extra fats. It's perfect for cooking lean meats, fish, and vegetables. Using a grill pan indoors can replicate the benefits of grilling when outdoor grilling isn't an option.
- Steamers: Steaming is another healthy cooking method that preserves the natural nutrients in vegetables without any need for cooking oil. It's particularly good for cooking delicate foods like fish and greens, which retain maximum flavor and texture through steaming.
- Slow Cookers and Pressure Cookers: These appliances are excellent for making stews, soups, and braised dishes, allowing flavors to develop deeply and naturally without the need for excess oil or fatty ingredients.

Cooking Techniques to Preserve Nutritional Integrity

- Steaming: This gentle cooking method keeps vegetables crisp, colorful, and nutrient-rich. It's particularly good for preparing vegetables like broccoli, spinach, and carrots, which can lose nutrients when overcooked by other methods.
- Grilling and Broiling: These methods allow fat to drip away from the food, reducing calorie intake and enhancing natural flavors. They are suitable for meats, fish, and even fruits and vegetables, providing a smoky flavor that can make meals more enjoyable without unhealthy additives.
- Baking and Roasting: Using an oven to bake or roast food can be a healthy alternative to frying. It requires minimal oil and can bring out natural flavors in foods especially when combined with herbs and spices.
- Sautéing with Water or Broth: Instead of using oil, try sautéing foods with a small amount of water or broth. This technique can help soften vegetables and unlock flavors in a healthier way.

Portion Control and Meal Balancing

- Portion Sizes: Understanding portion sizes is crucial. For example, a single serving of lean protein should be about the size of a deck of cards. Fill at least half of your plate with vegetables, a quarter with lean protein, and the remaining quarter with whole grains or another complex carbohydrate.
- Meal Balance: Always aim to include a variety of food groups in each meal. This ensures a balanced intake of carbohydrates, proteins, and fats, which supports overall metabolic health and liver function.
- Using Smaller Plates: To help manage portion sizes, use smaller plates for your meals. This can naturally encourage smaller servings and prevent overeating.

By equipping your kitchen with the right tools and adopting these cooking techniques, you can significantly improve the quality of your meals and their suitability for liver health. These strategies not only contribute to liver health but also enhance your overall nutritional intake, making your diet a powerful tool for maintaining wellness.

JOIN OUR CULINARY COMMUNITY!

Thank you for choosing the **Fatty Liver Diet Cookbook**. As you begin your journey of healthy eating and wellness, we are excited to join you in your culinary explorations aimed at supporting liver health.

Your insights are incredibly important to us and to the vibrant community of Fatty Liver Diet enthusiasts. We would deeply appreciate it if you could **share your experiences** by leaving a review on Amazon.

Here's how you can share your culinary stories:

1. Open the "Returns & Orders" section.

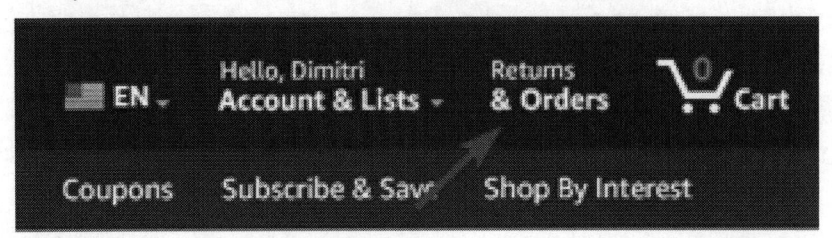

2. Select "Digital Orders".

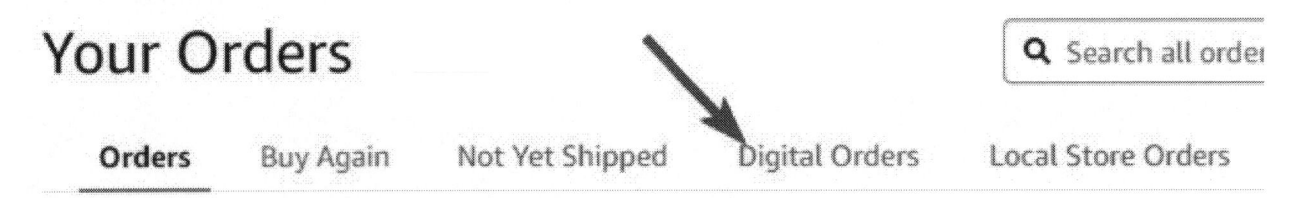

3. Find **Fatty Liver Diet Cookbook** and click "Write a product review".

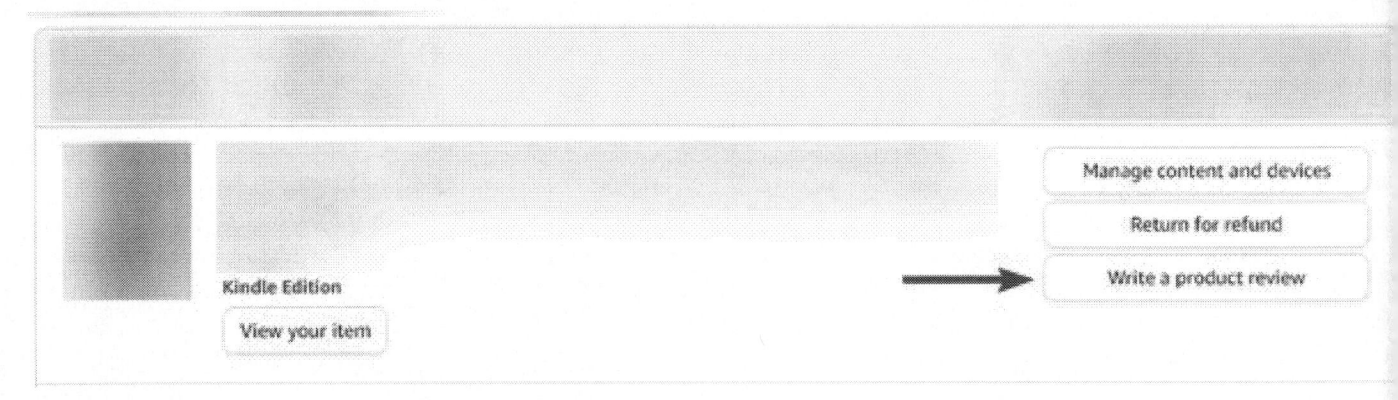

4. Leave your review about the book.

Whether it's your initial attempt at crafting a nutritious salad or a complete meal that supports liver health, your stories and feedback are crucial elements in our ongoing mission to enhance the experience of everyone following the Fatty Liver Diet. Thank you for contributing to our community and **helping us improve**!

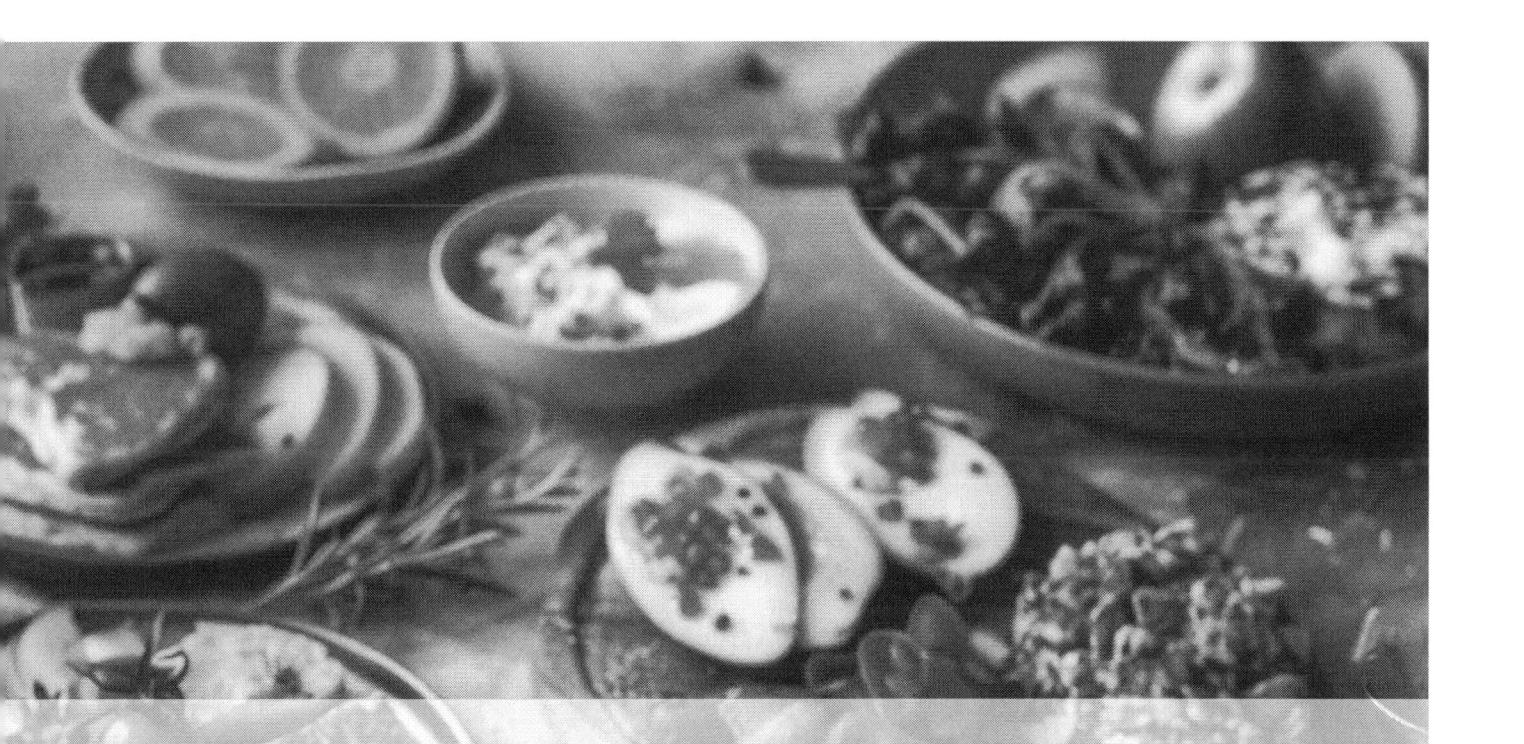

CHAPTER 3: NOURISHING BREAKFASTS TO START YOUR DAY RIGHT

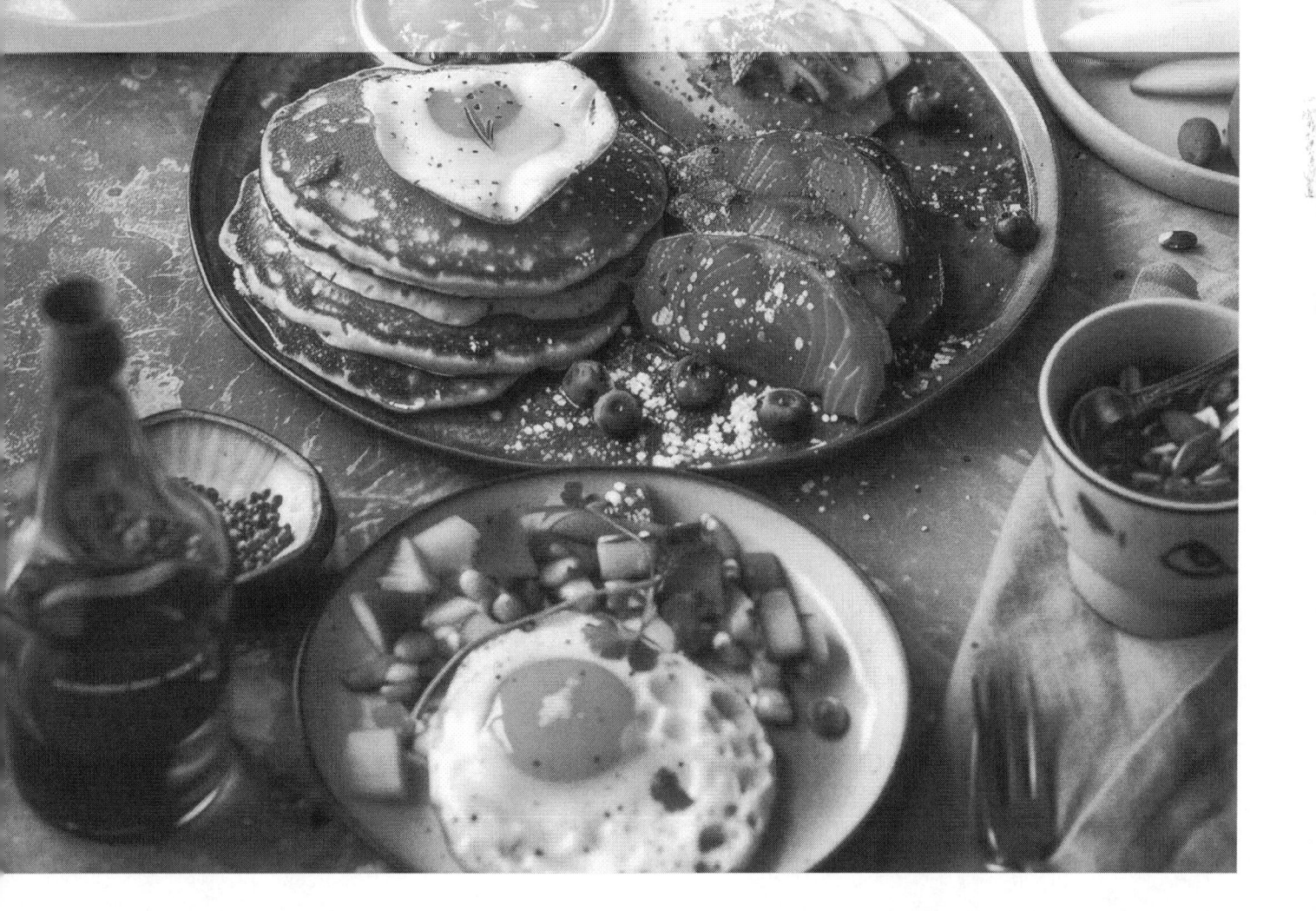

EASY-TO-FOLLOW, NUTRITIOUS BREAKFAST RECIPES

COTTAGE CHEESE PANCAKES WITH BLUEBERRIES

These cottage cheese pancakes with blueberries are a nutritious, tasty choice for breakfast, combining high protein, high fiber, and low-glycemic ingredients that are perfect for supporting liver health and overall well-being.

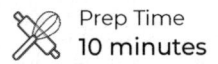

Prep Time: 10 minutes
Cooking Time: 15 minutes
Complexity: Beginner
Servings: 4
Ingredients: 8

EQUIPMENT NEEDED: Mixing bowl, non-stick skillet, measuring cups, measuring spoons, spatula
TAGS: High-protein, High-fiber, Low Glycemic, Heart-Healthy, Whole Foods, Low Sodium, Low Fat, Vitamin C rich

INGREDIENT LIST:

- 1 cup (236 ml) low-fat cottage cheese
- 2 large eggs
- 1/2 cup (120 ml) whole wheat flour
- 1/4 cup (60 ml) unsweetened almond milk
- 1 teaspoon (5 ml) baking powder
- 1/2 teaspoon (2.5 ml) vanilla extract
- 1 cup (236 ml) fresh blueberries
- Cooking spray for skillet

DIRECTIONS:

1. In a large mixing bowl, thoroughly mix the cottage cheese, eggs, almond milk, and vanilla extract until smooth.
2. Add the whole wheat flour and baking powder to the cottage cheese mixture and stir until just combined to avoid overmixing.
3. Carefully fold in the fresh blueberries to the batter to prevent them from crushing.
4. Preheat a non-stick skillet over medium heat and lightly coat with cooking spray.
5. Pour approximately 1/4 cup (60 ml) of batter for each pancake onto the hot skillet. Cook for about 2-3 minutes on each side until the pancakes are golden brown and fully cooked.
6. Serve the pancakes warm, optionally topped with additional fresh blueberries.

NUTRITION INFORMATION: (APPROXIMATE VALUES PER SERVING): Calories: 180 | Protein: 12g | Carbohydrates: 18g | Fats: 5g | Sodium: 200mg | Potassium: 125mg | Sugar: 4g | Cholesterol: 95mg

SMOKED SALMON AND AVOCADO TOAST

This Smoked Salmon and Avocado Toast offers a hearty, nutritious start to your day, packed with omega-3 fatty acids, healthy fats, and essential vitamins. It's perfect for those looking to support liver health while enjoying a flavorful breakfast.

Prep Time: 5 minutes
Cooking Time: 0 minutes
Complexity: Beginner
Servings: 4
Ingredients: 8

EQUIPMENT NEEDED: Knife, cutting board, toaster
TAGS: Heart-Healthy, High-Protein, Low Glycemic, High-Fiber, Low Sodium, Whole Foods

INGREDIENT LIST:

- 2 slices of whole grain bread (1 cup [236 ml])
- 4 ounces (113 g) smoked salmon
- 1 ripe avocado, sliced
- 1 tablespoon (15 ml) fresh lemon juice
- Fresh dill for garnish (optional)

DIRECTIONS:

1. Toast the whole grain bread slices to your preferred level of crispiness.
2. While the bread is toasting, slice the avocado and drizzle it with fresh lemon juice to enhance flavor and prevent browning.
3. Once the bread is toasted, evenly distribute the avocado slices on each piece of bread.
4. Top each slice with smoked salmon.
5. Garnish with fresh dill if desired, and serve immediately.

NUTRITION INFORMATION: (APPROXIMATE VALUES PER SERVING): Calories: 300 | Protein: 21g | Carbohydrates: 30g | Fats: 12g | Sodium: 450mg | Potassium: 500mg | Sugar: 3g | Cholesterol: 30mg

VEGAN TOFU SCRAMBLE WITH SPINACH AND TOMATOES

Start your day with this nutrient-rich Vegan Tofu Scramble, combining the goodness of tofu, spinach, and tomatoes. It's a perfect meal for maintaining a healthy liver and providing sustained energy throughout the day.

Prep Time: 10 minutes **Cooking Time:** 10 minutes **Complexity:** Beginner **Servings:** 2 **Ingredients:** 7

EQUIPMENT NEEDED: Skillet, spatula, knife, cutting board
TAGS: Vegan, Whole Foods, High-protein, High-fiber, Low Sodium, Low Glycemic, Heart-Healthy, Gluten-Free, Low Fat, Vitamin C rich

INGREDIENT LIST:

- 14 oz (400 g) firm tofu, drained and crumbled
- 1 cup (30 g) fresh spinach, roughly chopped
- 1 medium tomato, diced
- 1/4 cup (60 ml) nutritional yeast
- 1/2 teaspoon (2.5 ml) turmeric powder
- 2 tablespoons (30 ml) olive oil
- Salt and pepper to taste (minimal salt for low sodium)

DIRECTIONS:

1. Heat the olive oil in a skillet over medium heat.
2. Add the crumbled tofu and turmeric powder to the skillet, stirring to combine. Cook for about 5 minutes or until the tofu starts to turn golden.
3. Stir in the nutritional yeast for a cheesy flavor and added nutrients.
4. Add the chopped spinach and diced tomato to the skillet, cooking until the spinach wilts and the tomatoes are heated through, about 3-4 minutes.
5. Season with a minimal amount of salt and pepper to maintain a low sodium content.
6. Serve hot, garnished with additional fresh herbs if desired.

NUTRITION INFORMATION: (APPROXIMATE VALUES PER SERVING): Calories: 250 | Protein: 19g | Carbohydrates: 10g | Fats: 15g | Sodium: 200mg | Potassium: 300mg | Sugar: 3g | Cholesterol: 0mg

PEAR AND WALNUT OATMEAL

This Pear and Walnut Oatmeal is a heartwarming start to your day, combining the sweetness of pears with the crunch of walnuts in a fiber-rich meal that supports digestive health and liver function.

Prep Time: 5 minutes **Cooking Time:** 10 minutes **Complexity:** Beginner **Servings:** 2 **Ingredients:** 6

EQUIPMENT NEEDED: Pot, spoon, knife, cutting board
TAGS: Whole Foods, Vegetarian, High-fiber, Low Sodium, Heart-Healthy, Low Glycemic

INGREDIENT LIST:

- 1 cup (90 g) rolled oats
- 1 1/2 cups (355 ml) water or unsweetened almond milk
- 1 ripe pear, cored and chopped
- 1/4 cup (30 g) walnuts, chopped
- 1/2 teaspoon (2.5 ml) ground cinnamon
- 1 tablespoon (15 ml) ground flaxseed (optional for added fiber)

DIRECTIONS:

1. In a small pot, bring the water or almond milk to a boil.
2. Add the rolled oats and simmer on low heat for about 5 minutes, stirring occasionally until the oats are soft.
3. Stir in the chopped pear, walnuts, and cinnamon, cooking for another 2-3 minutes until the pear is tender.
4. Remove from heat and let sit for a couple of minutes to thicken. Stir in the ground flaxseed if using.
5. Serve warm, garnished with additional cinnamon or a drizzle of honey if desired for natural sweetness.

NUTRITION INFORMATION: (APPROXIMATE VALUES PER SERVING): Calories: 295 | Protein: 7g | Carbohydrates: 45g | Fats: 10g | Sodium: 30mg | Potassium: 200mg | Sugar: 10g | Cholesterol: 0mg

SPICED PUMPKIN PORRIDGE

This Spiced Pumpkin Porridge is a warming, nutritious breakfast option filled with fiber and essential nutrients. It perfectly embodies the spirit of fall and supports liver health with its whole food ingredients and low glycemic profile.

Prep Time: 5 minutes
Cooking Time: 15 minutes
Complexity: Beginner
Servings: 2
Ingredients: 8

EQUIPMENT NEEDED: Pot, spoon, measuring cups, measuring spoons

TAGS: Whole Foods, Vegan, High-fiber, Low Glycemic, Low Sodium, Low Fat, Vitamin A rich

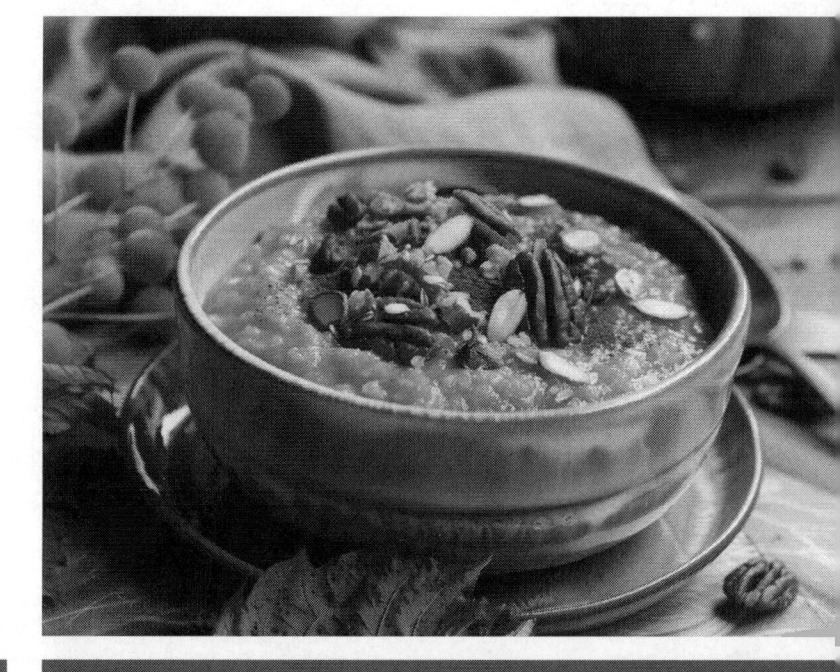

INGREDIENT LIST:

- 1/2 cup (120 ml) rolled oats
- 1 cup (236 ml) unsweetened almond milk
- 1/2 cup (120 ml) pumpkin puree
- 1/4 teaspoon (1.25 ml) ground cinnamon
- 1/8 teaspoon (0.625 ml) ground nutmeg
- 1/8 teaspoon (0.625 ml) ground ginger
- 1 tablespoon (15 ml) chia seeds
- 1 tablespoon (15 ml) maple syrup (optional)

DIRECTIONS:

1. Combine the rolled oats and almond milk in a pot over medium heat.
2. Bring the mixture to a boil, then reduce the heat and simmer for 5 minutes, stirring occasionally.
3. Stir in the pumpkin puree, cinnamon, nutmeg, ginger, and chia seeds. Continue to cook for another 5-10 minutes until the porridge has thickened to your liking.
4. Remove from heat and stir in maple syrup if using for a touch of sweetness.
5. Serve the porridge warm, and top with additional cinnamon or a sprinkle of nuts if desired.

NUTRITION INFORMATION: (APPROXIMATE VALUES PER SERVING): Calories: 180 | Protein: 6g | Carbohydrates: 27g | Fats: 4.5g | Sodium: 30mg | Potassium: 200mg | Sugar: 6g (only if maple syrup is used) | Cholesterol: 0mg

VEGETABLE HASH WITH POACHED EGG

This hearty Vegetable Hash with Poached Egg is a flavorful and nutritious breakfast option that offers a perfect mix of protein, fiber, and healthy fats, ideal for supporting liver health and maintaining a balanced diet.

- **Prep Time:** 10 minutes
- **Cooking Time:** 20 minutes
- **Complexity:** Intermediate
- **Servings:** 2
- **Ingredients:** 8

EQUIPMENT NEEDED: Skillet, pot, slotted spoon, knife, cutting board
TAGS: Whole Foods, Heart-Healthy, High-protein, High-fiber, Low Sodium, Gluten-Free, Low Glycemic

INGREDIENT LIST:

- 1 medium sweet potato, peeled and diced (1 cup [236 ml])
- 1/2 red bell pepper, diced
- 1/2 green bell pepper, diced
- 1 small onion, diced
- 2 cloves garlic, minced
- 2 large eggs
- 2 tablespoons (30 ml) olive oil
- Salt and pepper to taste (minimal salt for low sodium)

DIRECTIONS:

1. Heat the olive oil in a large skillet over medium heat. Add the diced sweet potato and cook for about 10 minutes, stirring occasionally, until they begin to soften.
2. Add the diced onions, red and green bell peppers, and garlic to the skillet. Continue to cook for another 8-10 minutes until all the vegetables are tender and lightly browned.
3. While the vegetables are cooking, bring a pot of water to a gentle simmer. Crack each egg into a small bowl and gently slide them into the simmering water one at a time. Poach the eggs for about 3-4 minutes until the whites are set but the yolks remain runny.
4. Season the vegetable hash with minimal salt and pepper to taste. Divide the vegetable hash between two plates, and carefully place a poached egg on top of each serving.
5. Serve immediately, garnished with fresh herbs like parsley or chives if desired.

NUTRITION INFORMATION: (APPROXIMATE VALUES PER SERVING): Calories: 320 | Protein: 11g | Carbohydrates: 35g | Fats: 16g | Sodium: 200mg | Potassium: 850mg | Sugar: 8g | Cholesterol: 186mg

WALNUT AND PEAR OAT BAKE

This Walnut and Pear Oat Bake is a delightful, warm breakfast dish that combines the heartiness of oats with the natural sweetness of pears and the crunchy texture of walnuts, making it an ideal meal for those on a fatty liver diet.

- **Prep Time:** 10 minutes
- **Cooking Time:** 25 minutes
- **Complexity:** Beginner
- **Servings:** 4
- **Ingredients:** 7

EQUIPMENT NEEDED: Mixing bowl, baking dish, measuring cups, measuring spoons, oven
TAGS: Whole Foods, Heart-Healthy, High-fiber, Low Sodium, Low Glycemic, Vegetarian, Gluten-Free

INGREDIENT LIST:

- 2 cups (190 g) gluten-free rolled oats, 1 large pear, cored and sliced (1 cup [236 ml])
- 1/2 cup (60 g) chopped walnuts
- 1 tsp (5 ml) ground cinnamon
- 2 cups (470 ml) unsweetened almond milk, 1/4 cup (60 ml) maple syrup (optional, depending on desired sweetness)
- 2 tbsp (30 ml) ground flaxseed (to add omega-3 fatty acids and fiber)

DIRECTIONS:

1. Preheat your oven to 375°F (190°C).
2. In a mixing bowl, combine the rolled oats, ground cinnamon, and ground flaxseed.
3. Stir in the unsweetened almond milk and maple syrup (if using) until well-mixed.
4. Fold in the chopped walnuts and sliced pears, mixing gently to distribute evenly.
5. Pour the mixture into a greased baking dish.
6. Bake in the preheated oven for 25 minutes, or until the top is golden and the oats are set.
7. Allow to cool slightly before serving. This dish can be enjoyed warm or at room temperature.

NUTRITION INFORMATION: (APPROXIMATE VALUES PER SERVING): Calories: 290 | Protein: 8g | Carbohydrates: 45g | Fats: 10g | Sodium: 30mg | Potassium: 200mg | Sugar: 12g (natural and added sugars) | Cholesterol: 0mg

SALMON AND AVOCADO TOAST

This Salmon and Avocado Toast combines healthy fats, lean protein, and whole grains to create a nourishing and satisfying breakfast option that supports liver health and cardiovascular wellness.

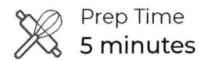

Prep Time: 5 minutes
Cooking Time: 5 minutes
Complexity: Beginner
Servings: 2
Ingredients: 5

EQUIPMENT NEEDED: Toaster, knife, cutting board, bowl
TAGS: Heart-healthy, High-protein, High-fiber, Low Sodium, Whole Foods, Gluten-Free

INGREDIENT LIST:

- 2 slices of gluten-free whole-grain bread
- 4 oz (113 g) smoked salmon
- 1 ripe avocado
- 1 tablespoon (15 ml) fresh lemon juice
- Fresh dill for garnish (optional)
- Black pepper to taste

DIRECTIONS:

1. Toast the gluten-free whole-grain bread slices to your desired level of crispiness.
2. In a bowl, mash the avocado with the fresh lemon juice and a pinch of black pepper.
3. Spread the mashed avocado evenly on the toasted bread slices.
4. Layer the smoked salmon over the avocado.
5. Garnish with fresh dill, if using, and serve immediately for the best flavor and texture.

NUTRITION INFORMATION: (APPROXIMATE VALUES PER SERVING): Calories: 300 | Protein: 20g | Carbohydrates: 30g | Fats: 15g | Sodium: 200mg | Potassium: 500mg | Sugar: 2g | Cholesterol: 20mg

QUINOA AND APPLE BREAKFAST BOWL

This Quinoa and Apple Breakfast Bowl is a wholesome and hearty start to your day, providing a perfect blend of protein, fiber, and healthy fats to support liver health and sustain energy levels.

Prep Time: 5 minutes
Cooking Time: 15 minutes
Complexity: Beginner
Servings: 2
Ingredients: 7

EQUIPMENT NEEDED: Pot, bowl, knife, cutting board
TAGS: Whole Foods, Heart-Healthy, High-fiber, Low Sodium, Vegetarian, Gluten-Free, High-protein, Low Glycemic

INGREDIENT LIST:

- 1/2 cup (95 g) quinoa, rinsed
- 1 cup (240 ml) water
- 1 medium apple, cored and chopped
- 1/2 teaspoon (2.5 ml) cinnamon
- 1/4 cup (30 g) walnuts, chopped
- 1 tablespoon (15 ml) chia seeds
- 1/4 cup (60 ml) almond milk (or any other plant-based milk)

DIRECTIONS:

1. Combine the quinoa and water in a pot and bring to a boil. Reduce heat to low, cover, and simmer until the quinoa is cooked and water is absorbed, about 15 minutes.
2. While the quinoa is cooking, chop the apple into bite-sized pieces.
3. Once the quinoa is cooked, fluff it with a fork and transfer it to a mixing bowl.
4. Stir in the almond milk, cinnamon, and chia seeds into the cooked quinoa.
5. Add the chopped apples and walnuts to the quinoa mixture and mix well.
6. Serve the breakfast bowl warm, or if preferred, it can also be enjoyed cold.

NUTRITION INFORMATION: (APPROXIMATE VALUES PER SERVING): Calories: 315 | Protein: 9g | Carbohydrates: 45g | Fats: 12g | Sodium: 30mg | Potassium: 400mg | Sugar: 10g | Cholesterol: 0mg

GRILLED CHICKEN AND AVOCADO WRAP

This Grilled Chicken and Avocado Wrap is a nutritious and satisfying breakfast option, combining lean protein from chicken, healthy fats from avocado, and whole grains from the wrap. It's designed to support liver health while aligning with the principles of a fatty liver diet.

Prep Time: 10 minutes
Cooking Time: 10 minutes
Complexity: Beginner
Servings: 2
Ingredients: 7

EQUIPMENT NEEDED: Grill pan, knife, cutting board, bowl, mixing spoon
TAGS: Whole Foods, Heart-Healthy, High-protein, Low Sodium, High-fiber

INGREDIENT LIST:

- 2 whole grain wraps (gluten-free if needed)
- 6 ounces (170 g) chicken breast, thinly sliced
- 1 ripe avocado, mashed
- 1/2 cup (30 g) fresh spinach leaves
- 1 small tomato, sliced
- 1 tablespoon (15 ml) olive oil
- Salt and pepper to taste (minimal salt for low sodium)

DIRECTIONS:

1. Heat the grill pan over medium heat and brush with olive oil.
2. Season the chicken slices with minimal salt and pepper, then grill them for about 5 minutes on each side or until fully cooked and slightly charred.
3. Warm the whole grain wraps in the microwave for 10-20 seconds to make them pliable.
4. Spread the mashed avocado evenly on each wrap.
5. Lay the grilled chicken slices over the avocado.
6. Add fresh spinach leaves and tomato slices on top of the chicken.
7. Roll up the wraps tightly, cut them in half, and serve immediately.

NUTRITION INFORMATION: (APPROXIMATE VALUES PER SERVING): Calories: 400 | Protein: 30g | Carbohydrates: 35g | Fats: 18g | Sodium: 200mg | Potassium: 800mg | Sugar: 3g | Cholesterol: 70mg

---

ALMOND BUTTER AND BANANA OATMEAL

This Almond Butter and Banana Oatmeal is a hearty, nutritious breakfast option packed with fiber, protein, and healthy fats. It's designed to keep you full and energized while supporting liver health and maintaining balanced blood sugar levels.

Prep Time: 5 minutes
Cooking Time: 10 minutes
Complexity: Beginner
Servings: 2
Ingredients: 6

EQUIPMENT NEEDED: Pot, spoon, bowls
TAGS: Whole Foods, Heart-Healthy, High-fiber, Low Sodium, Vegetarian, High-protein

INGREDIENT LIST:

- 1 cup (90 g) rolled oats
- 2 cups (480 ml) water or low-fat milk
- 1 medium banana, sliced
- 2 tablespoons (32 g) almond butter
- 1/2 teaspoon (2.5 ml) cinnamon
- 1 tablespoon (15 ml) chia seeds (optional for extra fiber)

DIRECTIONS:

1. In a medium pot, bring the water or milk to a boil.
2. Add the rolled oats and reduce heat to a simmer, cooking for about 5 minutes, stirring occasionally, until the oats are soft.
3. Remove the pot from heat and stir in the almond butter and cinnamon until fully combined.
4. Divide the oatmeal into bowls.
5. Top each bowl with sliced banana and a sprinkle of chia seeds if using.
6. Serve warm, and enjoy a comforting and filling breakfast.

NUTRITION INFORMATION: (APPROXIMATE VALUES PER SERVING): Calories: 350 | Protein: 12g | Carbohydrates: 50g | Fats: 14g | Sodium: 30mg | Potassium: 450mg | Sugar: 12g (natural sugars from banana and almond butter) | Cholesterol: 0mg

MIXED BERRY WHOLE GRAIN PORRIDGE

This Mixed Berry Whole Grain Porridge is a delightful and nutritious breakfast that combines whole grains with a colorful mix of berries, providing a fiber-rich, low-fat meal to start your day, perfect for supporting liver health and overall wellness.

Prep Time: 5 minutes
Cooking Time: 15 minutes
Complexity: Beginner
Servings: 2
Ingredients: 6

EQUIPMENT NEEDED: Pot, wooden spoon, bowls, measuring cups

TAGS: Whole Foods, Heart-Healthy, High-fiber, Low Sodium, Vegetarian, High-protein, Low Fat, Sugar-Free, Vitamin C rich

INGREDIENT LIST:

- 1/2 cup (90 g) whole grain oats or a mix of grains like barley, millet, and quinoa
- 2 cups (480 ml) water or low-fat milk
- 1/2 cup (75 g) mixed berries (strawberries, blueberries, raspberries), fresh or frozen
- 1 tablespoon (15 ml) ground flaxseed
- 1 teaspoon (5 ml) cinnamon
- Optional: natural sweeteners such as stevia or a drizzle of honey (omit for a strictly sugar-free diet)

DIRECTIONS:

1. In a medium-sized pot, bring the water or milk to a boil. Add the whole grains and reduce the heat to a simmer.
2. Cook the grains according to package instructions, usually about 10-15 minutes, until they are soft and have absorbed most of the liquid.
3. Stir in the ground flaxseed and cinnamon during the last few minutes of cooking.
4. Once the porridge is cooked, remove from heat and let it sit for a couple of minutes to thicken.
5. Gently fold in the mixed berries, allowing the heat of the porridge to slightly soften them.
6. Serve the porridge warm. If desired, sweeten with a small amount of stevia or a drizzle of honey.

NUTRITION INFORMATION: (APPROXIMATE VALUES PER SERVING): Calories: 200 | Protein: 8g | Carbohydrates: 38g | Fats: 3g | Sodium: 30mg | Potassium: 200mg | Sugar: 6g (natural sugars from berries, additional if honey is used) | Cholesterol: 0mg

SPINACH AND EGG WHITE OMELETTE

This Spinach and Egg White Omelette is a light and nutritious breakfast option, rich in protein and packed with vitamins. It's perfect for those following a fatty liver diet, providing essential nutrients while keeping calorie and fat intake low.

Prep Time: 5 minutes
Cooking Time: 5 minutes
Complexity: Beginner
Servings: 1
Ingredients: 5

EQUIPMENT NEEDED: Non-stick skillet, mixing bowl, whisk, spatula

TAGS: Heart-healthy, High-protein, Low Sodium, Low Fat, High-fiber, Gluten-Free, Vegetarian, Sugar-Free, Vitamin A rich, Vitamin C rich

INGREDIENT LIST:

- 3/4 cup (180 ml) egg whites
- 1 cup (30 g) fresh spinach, chopped
- 1 small onion, finely chopped
- 1/4 teaspoon (1.25 ml) black pepper
- 1 tablespoon (15 ml) olive oil

DIRECTIONS:

1. Heat the olive oil in a non-stick skillet over medium heat.
2. Sauté the chopped onion in the skillet until it becomes translucent, about 2 minutes.
3. Add the chopped spinach to the skillet and cook until it wilts, approximately 1-2 minutes.
4. In a mixing bowl, whisk the egg whites with black pepper.
5. Pour the egg whites over the sautéed spinach and onion in the skillet.
6. Cook the omelette for about 3 minutes or until the egg whites are set and fully cooked. Use a spatula to fold the omelette in half.
7. Slide the omelette onto a plate and serve hot.

NUTRITION INFORMATION: (APPROXIMATE VALUES PER SERVING): Calories: 180 | Protein: 20g | Carbohydrates: 5g | Fats: 8g | Sodium: 170mg | Potassium: 300mg | Sugar: 2g | Cholesterol: 0mg

SPECIAL SECTION: QUICK BREAKFASTS FOR BUSY MORNINGS

MANGO AND COCONUT CHIA PUDDING

This Mango and Coconut Chia Pudding is a refreshing, nutritious start to your day, offering a blend of high fiber, heart-healthy fats, and low-glycemic ingredients ideal for a fatty liver diet.

Prep Time: 15 minutes **Cooking Time:** 0 minutes **Complexity:** Beginner **Servings:** 4 **Ingredients:** 6

EQUIPMENT NEEDED: Mixing bowl, whisk, measuring cups, measuring spoons, refrigerator

TAGS: Whole Foods, Vegan, Low Glycemic, Heart-Healthy, Gluten-Free, Dairy-Free, High-Fiber, Low Sodium, Low Fat, Low Calorie, Vitamin C rich

INGREDIENT LIST:

- 1 cup (236 ml) unsweetened almond milk
- 1/4 cup (59 ml) chia seeds
- 1/2 cup (118 ml) coconut yogurt (dairy-free)
- 1 ripe mango, peeled and diced (high in Vitamin C)
- 2 tablespoons (30 ml) shredded unsweetened coconut
- 1 tablespoon (15 ml) pure maple syrup (optional, can be omitted for sugar-free needs)

DIRECTIONS:

1. In a mixing bowl, whisk together the almond milk, coconut yogurt, and chia seeds until well combined.
2. If using, stir in the maple syrup to sweeten the mixture.
3. Divide the mixture evenly into four serving dishes or one large container.
4. Cover and refrigerate overnight to allow the chia seeds to swell and the pudding to thicken.
5. Before serving, top each pudding with diced mango and a sprinkle of shredded coconut.

NUTRITION INFORMATION: (APPROXIMATE VALUES PER SERVING): Calories: 150 | Protein: 3g | Carbohydrates: 19g | Fats: 7g | Sodium: 55mg | Potassium: 150mg | Sugar: 10g (natural sugars from fruit, less if maple syrup is omitted) | Cholesterol: 0mg

BEETROOT AND CARROT JUICE CLEANSE

This Beetroot and Carrot Juice is a vibrant, nutrient-packed drink, perfect for detoxifying and supporting liver health while being naturally low in fats and sugars.

Prep Time: 10 minutes **Cooking Time:** 0 minutes **Complexity:** Beginner **Servings:** 2 **Ingredients:** 4

EQUIPMENT NEEDED: Juicer, knife, cutting board, measuring cups

TAGS: Whole Foods, Vegan, Low Glycemic, Heart-Healthy, Gluten-Free, Dairy-Free, High-Fiber, Low Sodium, Low Fat, Low Calorie, Vitamin A rich, Vitamin C rich

INGREDIENT LIST:

- 2 medium beetroots (beets), peeled and quartered (1 cup [236 ml])
- 4 large carrots, peeled and cut into chunks (1 cup [236 ml])
- 1 large apple, cored and quartered (optional for sweetness)
- 1-inch piece of fresh ginger, peeled (2.5 cm)

DIRECTIONS:

1. Prepare all the ingredients by washing, peeling, and cutting them into sizes suitable for your juicer.
2. Start with the harder vegetables first. Juice the beetroots and carrots alternately with the apple and ginger to help push through all the fibrous material.
3. Once all the ingredients have been juiced, stir the mixture to combine.
4. Serve the juice immediately for best taste and nutrient retention, or store in a sealed container in the refrigerator for up to 24 hours.

NUTRITION INFORMATION: (APPROXIMATE VALUES PER SERVING): Calories: 95 | Protein: 2g | Carbohydrates: 22g | Fats: 0.3g | Sodium: 77mg | Potassium: 687mg | Sugar: 14g (natural sugars from vegetables and apple) | Cholesterol: 0mg

BROCCOLI AND FETA CHEESE SCRAMBLE

This Broccoli and Feta Cheese Scramble is a nutrient-dense breakfast option that combines high-quality protein, fiber, and essential vitamins to support liver health and overall wellness.

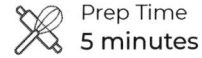

- **Prep Time:** 5 minutes
- **Cooking Time:** 10 minutes
- **Complexity:** Beginner
- **Servings:** 2
- **Ingredients:** 6

EQUIPMENT NEEDED: Skillet, spatula, knife, cutting board
TAGS: High-protein, High-fiber, Low Sodium, Low Glycemic, Heart-Healthy, Whole Foods, Vegetarian

INGREDIENT LIST:

- 1 cup (236 ml) of chopped fresh broccoli
- 4 large eggs
- 1/4 cup (59 ml) crumbled feta cheese (low-fat)
- 1 tablespoon (15 ml) olive oil
- Salt and pepper to taste (use minimal salt for low sodium)
- Fresh herbs (such as parsley or chives) for garnish (optional)

DIRECTIONS:

1. Heat the olive oil in a skillet over medium heat.
2. Add the chopped broccoli and sauté until it is bright green and tender, about 5 minutes.
3. In a bowl, beat the eggs and then pour them over the broccoli in the skillet.
4. Sprinkle the crumbled feta cheese over the eggs and broccoli. Stir gently to combine.
5. Cook until the eggs are set, about 5 minutes, stirring occasionally to create a scrambled texture.
6. Season with minimal salt and pepper to taste. Garnish with fresh herbs if desired.
7. Serve hot.

NUTRITION INFORMATION: (APPROXIMATE VALUES PER SERVING): Calories: 250 | Protein: 19g | Carbohydrates: 6g | Fats: 18g | Sodium: 320mg | Potassium: 340mg | Sugar: 2g | Cholesterol: 372mg

GREEN TEA YOGURT PARFAIT

This Green Tea Yogurt Parfait offers a refreshing and healthy start to your day, combining the antioxidant benefits of green tea with the probiotic richness of yogurt and the fiber of fresh fruits.

- **Prep Time:** 5 minutes
- **Cooking Time:** 0 minutes
- **Complexity:** Beginner
- **Servings:** 2
- **Ingredients:** 5

EQUIPMENT NEEDED: Mixing bowl, whisk, two parfait glasses or bowls, spoon
TAGS: Whole Foods, Heart-Healthy, High-fiber, Low Sodium, Low Glycemic, Gluten-Free, Vegetarian

INGREDIENT LIST:

- 1 cup (240 ml) low-fat Greek yogurt
- 1 teaspoon (5 ml) matcha green tea powder
- 1 tablespoon (15 ml) honey (optional, depending on desired sweetness)
- 1/2 cup (120 ml) fresh berries (blueberries, raspberries, or strawberries)
- 1/4 cup (30 g) granola (gluten-free if necessary)

DIRECTIONS:

1. In a mixing bowl, whisk the Greek yogurt with the matcha green tea powder until well combined. Add honey if desired for a touch of sweetness.
2. Layer half of the green tea yogurt mixture into two parfait glasses.
3. Add a layer of fresh berries on top of the yogurt in each glass.
4. Sprinkle half of the granola over the berries.
5. Repeat the layers with the remaining yogurt, berries, and granola.
6. Serve immediately or refrigerate until ready to serve for a chilled breakfast option.

NUTRITION INFORMATION: (APPROXIMATE VALUES PER SERVING): Calories: 180 | Protein: 12g | Carbohydrates: 18g | Fats: 6g | Sodium: 60mg | Potassium: 200mg | Sugar: 10g (natural and added, if honey is used) | Cholesterol: 10mg

CHIA SEED AND RASPBERRY PUDDING

This Chia Seed and Raspberry Pudding is a delightful and nutritious breakfast option, rich in omega-3 fatty acids, fiber, and antioxidants, making it ideal for supporting liver health and overall well-being.

Prep Time: 10 minutes | **Cooking Time:** 0 minutes | **Complexity:** Beginner | **Servings:** 2 | **Ingredients:** 5

EQUIPMENT NEEDED: Mixing bowl, whisk, two serving glasses or bowls, refrigerator
TAGS: Whole Foods, Vegan, Low Glycemic, Heart-Healthy, High-fiber, Low Sodium, Gluten-Free, Low Fat, Dairy-Free, Sugar-Free

INGREDIENT LIST:

- 1/4 cup (60 ml) chia seeds
- 1 cup (240 ml) unsweetened almond milk
- 1/2 teaspoon (2.5 ml) vanilla extract
- 1 cup (125 g) fresh raspberries
- Optional sweetener: 1 tablespoon (15 ml) of honey or agave syrup (omit for sugar-free diet)

DIRECTIONS:

1. In a mixing bowl, combine the chia seeds, almond milk, and vanilla extract. Whisk thoroughly to mix.
2. If using a sweetener, add honey or agave syrup to the mixture and whisk again to incorporate.
3. Divide the mixture evenly between two serving glasses or bowls.
4. Gently stir half of the raspberries into each serving.
5. Cover and refrigerate for at least 4 hours, or overnight, until the chia seeds have absorbed the liquid and the pudding has thickened.
6. Serve chilled, topped with additional raspberries or a sprinkle of crushed nuts for extra crunch.

NUTRITION INFORMATION: (APPROXIMATE VALUES PER SERVING): Calories: 180 | Protein: 4g | Carbohydrates: 20g | Fats: 10g | Sodium: 45mg | Potassium: 150mg | Sugar: 5g (natural sugars from raspberries, none if no sweetener is used) | Cholesterol: 0mg

WHOLE WHEAT PANCAKES WITH FRESH FRUIT

Enjoy a heart-healthy and fiber-rich start to your day with these whole wheat pancakes topped with a variety of fresh fruits. This simple yet delicious recipe provides a good balance of complex carbohydrates, protein, and healthy fats.

Prep Time: 10 minutes | **Cooking Time:** 10 minutes | **Complexity:** Beginner | **Servings:** 4 | **Ingredients:** 8

EQUIPMENT NEEDED: Mixing bowl, whisk, non-stick skillet or griddle, spatula, measuring cups, measuring spoons
TAGS: Whole Foods, Heart-Healthy, High-fiber, Low Sodium, Vegetarian

INGREDIENT LIST:

- 1 cup (120 g) whole wheat flour
- 1 tablespoon (15 ml) baking powder
- 1/4 teaspoon (1.25 ml) salt (optional, can omit for lower sodium)
- 1 cup (240 ml) low-fat milk or plant-based milk
- 1 large egg
- 2 tablespoons (30 ml) olive oil or melted unsalted butter
- 1 teaspoon (5 ml) vanilla extract
- 1 cup (150 g) mixed fresh fruits (blueberries, sliced strawberries, and banana slices)

DIRECTIONS:

1. In a large mixing bowl, whisk together the whole wheat flour, baking powder, and salt.
2. In another bowl, beat together the milk, egg, olive oil, and vanilla extract.
3. Pour the wet ingredients into the dry ingredients and stir until just combined; the batter should be slightly lumpy.
4. Heat a non-stick skillet or griddle over medium heat and lightly grease it with a little olive oil or cooking spray.
5. Pour 1/4 cup (60 ml) of batter for each pancake onto the skillet. Cook until bubbles form on the surface of the pancakes and the edges look set, about 2-3 minutes.
6. Flip the pancakes and cook for another 2-3 minutes on the other side until golden brown.
7. Serve the pancakes hot, topped with a generous amount of mixed fresh fruits.

NUTRITION INFORMATION: (APPROXIMATE VALUES PER SERVING): Calories: 250 | Protein: 8g | Carbohydrates: 38g | Fats: 9g | Sodium: 300mg (less if salt is omitted) | Potassium: 200mg | Sugar: 8g | Cholesterol: 55mg

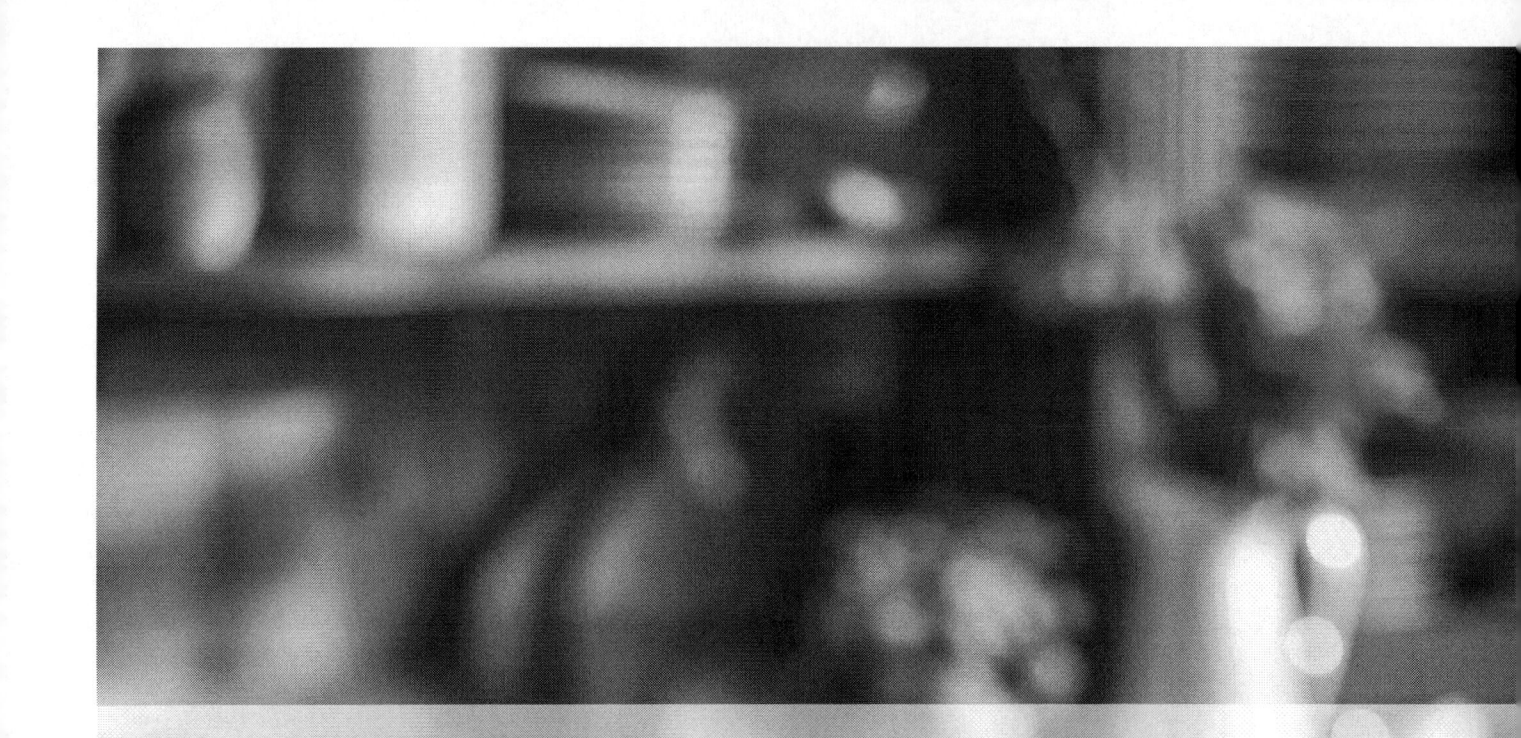

CHAPTER 4: LUNCHES TO LOVE

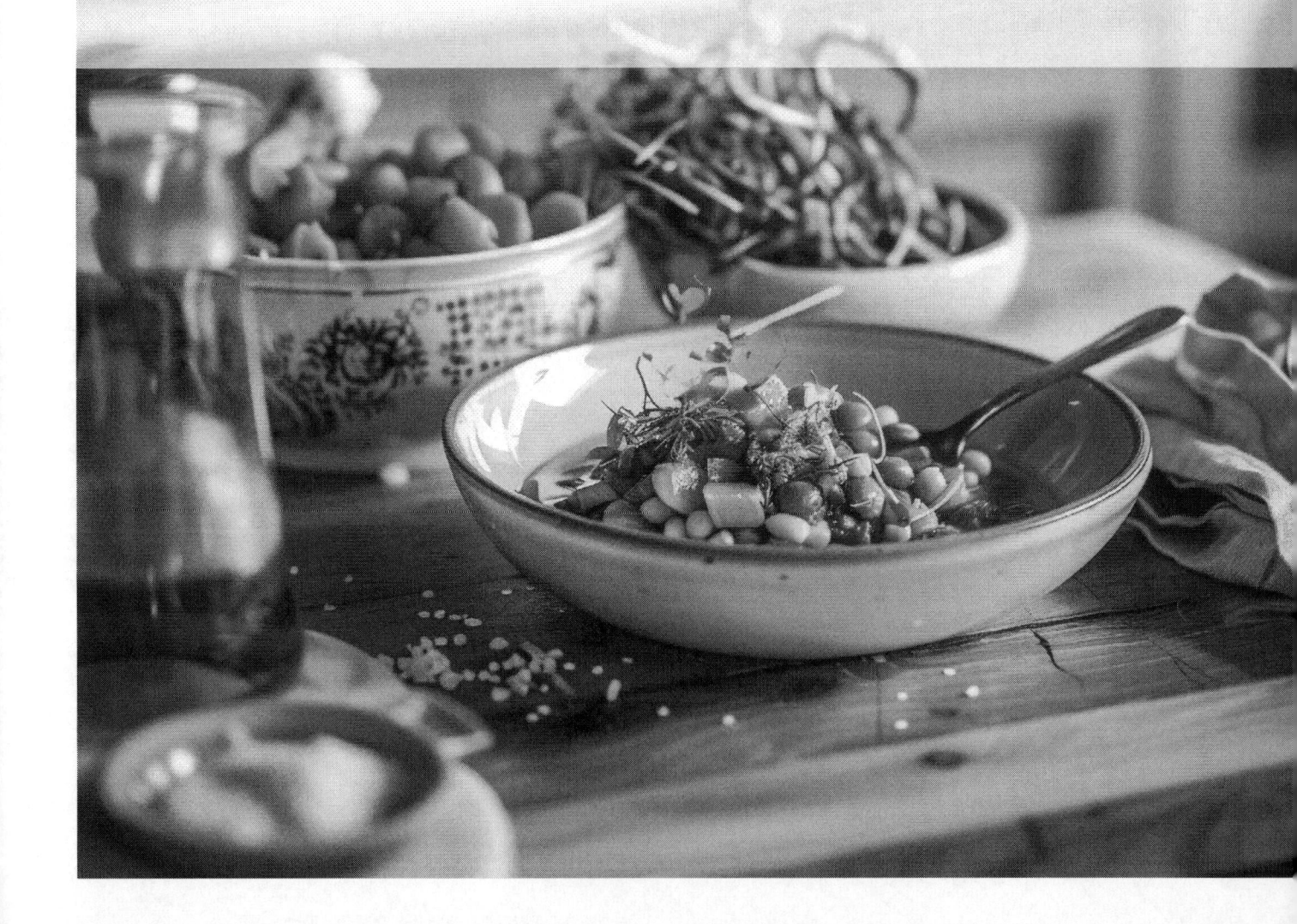

DELICIOUS AND HEALTHY LUNCH RECIPES

QUINOA TABBOULEH WITH CHICKPEAS

Quinoa Tabbouleh with Chickpeas is a fiber-rich and protein-packed dish that's perfect for breakfast. This version incorporates whole foods that align with fatty liver diet guidelines while delivering a refreshing and wholesome flavor.

Prep Time: 10 minutes
Cooking Time: 15 minutes
Complexity: Beginner
Servings: 4
Ingredients: 9

EQUIPMENT NEEDED: Pot, mixing bowl, spoon, knife, cutting board, fine mesh sieve

TAGS: Whole Foods, Heart-Healthy, High-protein, High-fiber, Low Sodium, Low Fat, Gluten-Free, Vegan, Low Glycemic, Vitamin C rich

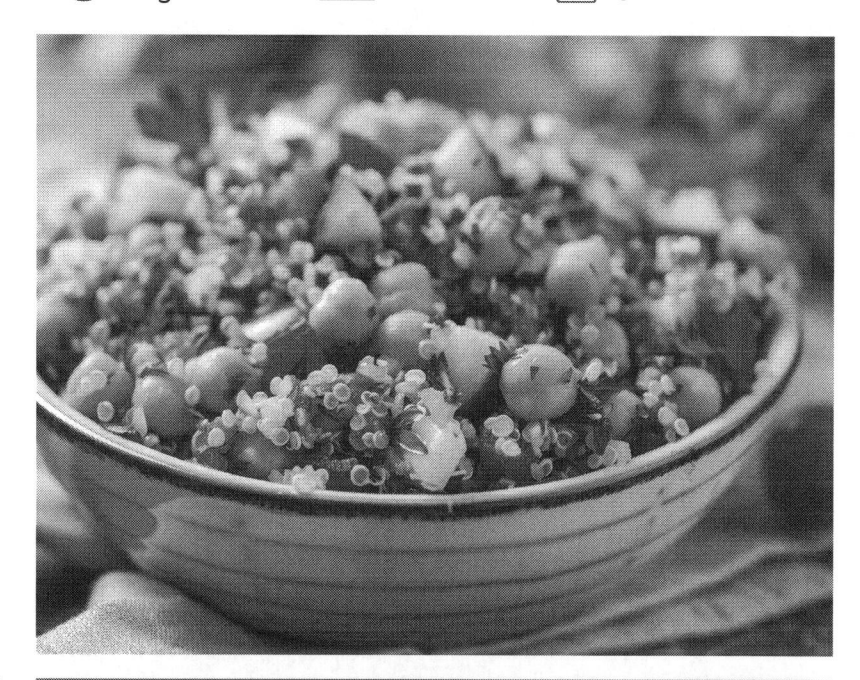

INGREDIENT LIST:

- 1 cup (180 g) quinoa, rinsed
- 2 cups (480 ml) water
- 1 cup (150 g) cooked chickpeas, rinsed and drained
- 1 cup (30 g) parsley, chopped
- 1/2 cup (75 g) tomatoes, diced
- 1/4 cup (30 g) cucumber, diced
- 2 tablespoons (30 ml) fresh lemon juice
- 2 tablespoons (30 ml) olive oil
- 1/4 teaspoon (1.25 ml) black pepper

DIRECTIONS:

1. In a pot, combine the quinoa and water. Bring to a boil over medium heat, then reduce to a simmer and cover. Cook for about 15 minutes until all the water is absorbed. Fluff with a fork and set aside to cool.
2. In a large mixing bowl, combine the cooked quinoa, chickpeas, parsley, tomatoes, and cucumber.
3. In a small bowl, whisk together the lemon juice, olive oil, and black pepper.
4. Pour the dressing over the quinoa mixture and gently toss until evenly coated.
5. Serve immediately or refrigerate for later use.

NUTRITION INFORMATION: (APPROXIMATE VALUES PER SERVING): Calories: 220 | Protein: 7g | Carbohydrates: 35g | Fats: 5g | Sodium: 80mg | Potassium: 350mg | Sugar: 3g | Cholesterol: 0mg

HEARTY MINESTRONE SOUP WITH WHOLE WHEAT PASTA

A warm, filling soup that combines whole wheat pasta with nutrient-rich vegetables, this Hearty Minestrone Soup is perfect for a satisfying breakfast. It's packed with fiber, vitamins, and lean proteins, adhering to the fatty liver diet guidelines.

Prep Time: 15 minutes
Cooking Time: 30 minutes
Complexity: Beginner
Servings: 6
Ingredients: 14

EQUIPMENT NEEDED: Large pot, knife, cutting board, spoon, ladle
TAGS: Heart-healthy, High-fiber, Low Sodium, Low Fat, Low Glycemic, Whole Foods, Vegetarian, Vitamin A rich, Vitamin C rich

INGREDIENT LIST:

- 1 tablespoon (15 ml) olive oil, 1 medium onion, diced, 2 garlic cloves, minced
- 1 medium carrot, diced, 1 stalk celery, diced
- 1 small zucchini, diced, 1 cup (200 g) canned, no-salt-added diced tomatoes
- 4 cups (950 ml) low-sodium vegetable broth, 1 cup (180 g) canned no-salt-added kidney beans, drained and rinsed
- 1 cup (150 g) whole wheat pasta (penne or elbow macaroni)
- 1 teaspoon (5 ml) dried oregano
- 1 teaspoon (5 ml) dried basil
- 2 cups (60 g) fresh spinach, chopped
- 1/4 teaspoon (1.25 ml) black pepper

DIRECTIONS:

1. In a large pot, heat olive oil over medium heat.
2. Add diced onion, minced garlic, diced carrot, and diced celery. Sauté for 5-6 minutes until softened.
3. Add the diced zucchini and cook for another 2 minutes.
4. Pour in the diced tomatoes and vegetable broth. Stir in oregano, basil, and black pepper.
5. Bring the mixture to a boil, then reduce to a simmer. Add the whole wheat pasta and cook for 10-12 minutes until al dente.
6. Add the kidney beans and spinach, stirring gently. Cook for another 5 minutes until the spinach wilts.
7. Taste and adjust the seasoning if needed.
8. Serve hot, garnished with fresh herbs if desired.

NUTRITION INFORMATION: (APPROXIMATE VALUES PER SERVING): Calories: 180 | Protein: 8g | Carbohydrates: 30g | Sodium: 150mg | Fats: 4g | Potassium: 400mg | Sugar: 6g | Cholesterol: 0mg

GRILLED HADDOCK WITH OLIVE TAPENADE

This Grilled Haddock with Olive Tapenade is a healthy and flavorful breakfast. Packed with lean protein from haddock and healthy fats from olives, it provides essential nutrients while being low in fat and sodium.

Prep Time: 10 minutes
Cooking Time: 15 minutes
Complexity: Beginner
Servings: 4
Ingredients: 8

EQUIPMENT NEEDED: Grill or grill pan, bowl, spoon, tongs
TAGS: Heart-healthy, High-protein, Low Glycemic, Whole Foods, Low Fat, Low Sodium, Gluten-Free, Vitamin D rich

INGREDIENT LIST:

- 4 haddock fillets (about 4 oz or 113 g each)
- 2 tablespoons (30 ml) olive oil, divided
- 1 teaspoon (5 ml) lemon zest
- 1/4 teaspoon (1.25 ml) black pepper
- 1/4 cup (60 g) pitted kalamata olives, chopped
- 1 tablespoon (15 ml) capers, rinsed and chopped
- 1 teaspoon (5 ml) lemon juice
- 2 tablespoons (30 ml) parsley, chopped

DIRECTIONS:

1. **Preheat Grill:** Preheat a grill or grill pan over medium-high heat.
2. **Season Haddock:** Rub the haddock fillets with 1 tablespoon of olive oil, lemon zest, and black pepper.
3. **Grill Haddock:** Grill the fillets for about 3-4 minutes per side or until the fish flakes easily with a fork. Transfer to a serving plate.
4. **Prepare Tapenade:** In a bowl, combine chopped olives, capers, lemon juice, parsley, and the remaining olive oil. Mix well.
5. **Top Haddock:** Spoon the olive tapenade over the grilled haddock fillets.
6. **Serve:** Serve the grilled haddock hot with a lemon wedge on the side, if desired.

NUTRITION INFORMATION: (APPROXIMATE VALUES PER SERVING): Calories: 180 | Protein: 25g | Carbohydrates: 2g | Sodium: 170mg | Fats: 8g | Potassium: 400mg | Sugar: 0g | Cholesterol: 40mg

CARROT AND GINGER PURÉE SOUP

A warm and comforting breakfast soup, this carrot and ginger purée offers a nutrient-rich and flavorful start to your day. It's packed with vitamins and is low in fat, ideal for the fatty liver diet.

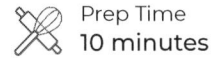

Prep Time: 10 minutes
Cooking Time: 25 minutes
Complexity: Beginner
Servings: 4
Ingredients: 9

EQUIPMENT NEEDED: Pot, immersion blender (or regular blender), spoon, knife, cutting board

TAGS: Whole Foods, Heart-Healthy, Low Glycemic, High-Fiber, Low Sodium, Low Fat, Gluten-Free, Vitamin A Rich, Vitamin C Rich, Dairy-Free, Vegan

INGREDIENT LIST:

- 1 tablespoon (15 ml) olive oil
- 1 medium onion, chopped
- 2 cloves garlic, minced
- 1-inch piece of fresh ginger, peeled and grated
- 6 medium carrots (about 1 lb or 450 g), peeled and chopped
- 4 cups (960 ml) low-sodium vegetable broth
- 1 teaspoon (5 ml) ground cumin
- Salt and pepper to taste
- Fresh cilantro for garnish

DIRECTIONS:

1. **Sauté Aromatics:** In a pot over medium heat, warm olive oil. Add chopped onion, minced garlic, and grated ginger. Sauté for 4-5 minutes until softened and fragrant.
2. **Add Carrots:** Add chopped carrots and cumin. Stir to combine and cook for 2 minutes.
3. **Simmer:** Pour in vegetable broth, cover the pot, and bring to a boil. Reduce heat to a simmer and cook for about 20 minutes or until carrots are tender.
4. **Purée:** Using an immersion blender (or regular blender in batches), blend the soup until smooth. Season with salt and pepper to taste.
5. **Garnish:** Ladle into bowls and garnish with fresh cilantro. Serve warm.

NUTRITION INFORMATION: (APPROXIMATE VALUES PER SERVING): Calories: 120 | Protein: 2g | Carbohydrates: 17g | Sodium: 200mg | Fats: 5g | Potassium: 420mg | Sugar: 6g | Cholesterol: 0mg

SPICED LENTIL STEW WITH COCONUT MILK

A warm and flavorful lentil stew simmered with aromatic spices and creamy coconut milk. This filling breakfast is packed with fiber, protein, and essential vitamins.

Prep Time: 15 minutes
Cooking Time: 30 minutes
Complexity: Beginner
Servings: 4
Ingredients: 12

EQUIPMENT NEEDED: Large pot, spoon, knife, cutting board, bowl

TAGS: Whole Foods, vegan, Heart-Healthy, gluten-free, dairy-free, High-protein, High-fiber, Low Glycemic, Low Sodium, low-fat, Vitamin A rich, Vitamin C rich

INGREDIENT LIST:

- 1 cup (200 g) dry red lentils, rinsed and drained,
- 1 tablespoon (15 ml) coconut oil
- 2 cloves garlic, minced
- 1-inch (2.5 cm) fresh ginger, grated, 1 teaspoon (5 g) ground cumin
- 1 teaspoon (5 g) ground coriander, 1/2 teaspoon (2.5 g) turmeric powder, 1 medium onion, diced
- 1 teaspoon (5 g) paprika
- 1 cup (240 ml) coconut milk
- 4 cups (960 ml) vegetable broth
- Fresh cilantro for garnish

DIRECTIONS:

1. **Prepare the Aromatics:** In a large pot, heat the coconut oil over medium heat. Add diced onion and sauté until translucent, about 3-4 minutes. Add minced garlic and grated ginger, and cook for another minute until fragrant.
2. **Add Spices:** Stir in ground cumin, coriander, turmeric, and paprika. Cook for 1 minute, allowing the spices to release their aroma. Combine Lentils: Add rinsed lentils to the pot and stir to coat with the spices.
3. **Simmer the Stew:** Pour in coconut milk and vegetable broth. Bring to a boil, then reduce the heat to a simmer. Cover the pot and cook for 25-30 minutes or until the lentils are tender.
4. **Garnish and Serve:** Season the stew with salt and pepper to taste. Serve hot, garnished with fresh cilantro.

NUTRITION INFORMATION: (APPROXIMATE VALUES PER SERVING): Calories: 320 | Protein: 12g | Carbohydrates: 36g | Sodium: 380mg | Fats: 14g | Potassium: 520mg | Sugar: 3g | Cholesterol: 0mg

TUNA AND WHITE BEAN SALAD

A quick and nourishing salad perfect for breakfast. This tuna and white bean combination is high in protein, low in fat, and delivers vitamins and minerals to start your day right.

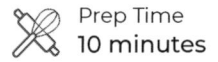

Prep Time: 10 minutes
Cooking Time: 0 minutes
Complexity: Beginner
Servings: 4
Ingredients: 10

EQUIPMENT NEEDED: Bowl, spoon, knife, cutting board

TAGS: Whole Foods, Heart-Healthy, Low Glycemic, High-Protein, High-Fiber, Low Sodium, Low Fat, Gluten-Free, Dairy-Free, Vitamin C Rich

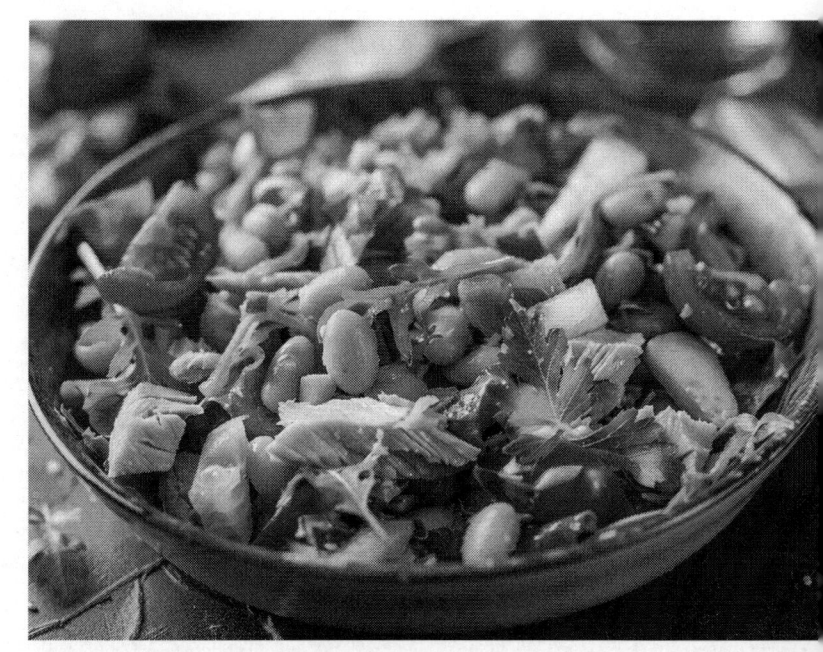

INGREDIENT LIST:

- 2 (5-ounce or 142-gram) cans of tuna packed in water, drained
- 1 (15-ounce or 425-gram) can of cannellini beans, drained and rinsed
- 1 medium cucumber, diced
- 1 small red onion, finely chopped
- 1 cup (100 g) cherry tomatoes, halved
- 1/4 cup (60 ml) fresh parsley, chopped
- 2 tablespoons (30 ml) lemon juice
- 2 tablespoons (30 ml) extra-virgin olive oil
- Salt and pepper to taste
- Fresh basil leaves for garnish

DIRECTIONS:

1. **Prepare Salad Base:** In a large bowl, combine drained tuna, cannellini beans, diced cucumber, chopped onion, and halved cherry tomatoes.
2. **Season Salad:** Add lemon juice, olive oil, chopped parsley, salt, and pepper to taste. Mix gently but thoroughly to combine.
3. **Garnish and Serve:** Divide the salad among plates and garnish with fresh basil leaves. Serve immediately or refrigerate for later.

NUTRITION INFORMATION: (APPROXIMATE VALUES PER SERVING): Calories: 230 | Protein: 20g | Carbohydrates: 15g | Sodium: 230mg | Fats: 8g | Potassium: 550mg | Sugar: 3g | Cholesterol: 20mg

GARLIC ROASTED TROUT WITH BRUSSELS SPROUTS

A wholesome breakfast combining the rich, savory flavors of garlic-seasoned trout with the earthy taste of roasted Brussels sprouts. Packed with protein, fiber, and essential vitamins, this meal is a nutritious way to start the day.

- **Prep Time:** 15 minutes
- **Cooking Time:** 20 minutes
- **Complexity:** Beginner
- **Servings:** 4
- **Ingredients:** 8

EQUIPMENT NEEDED: Baking sheet, parchment paper, small bowl, spoon, knife, cutting board

TAGS: Whole Foods, Heart-Healthy, gluten-free, dairy-free, High-protein, High-fiber, Low Glycemic, Low Sodium, low-fat, Vitamin D rich, Vitamin C rich

INGREDIENT LIST:

- 4 trout fillets, 4-6 oz each (115-170 g)
- 1 lb (450 g) Brussels sprouts, trimmed and halved
- 2 tablespoons (30 ml) extra-virgin olive oil
- 3 cloves garlic, minced
- 1 teaspoon (5 g) paprika
- 1 teaspoon (5 g) dried oregano
- 1 teaspoon (5 g) black pepper
- Salt to taste

DIRECTIONS:

1. **Preheat Oven:** Preheat the oven to 400°F (200°C). Line a baking sheet with parchment paper.
2. **Prepare Brussels Sprouts:** In a small bowl, combine 1 tablespoon olive oil, minced garlic, paprika, oregano, black pepper, and salt. Toss Brussels sprouts in the mixture until well coated. Arrange them on the prepared baking sheet, cut side down.
3. **Roast Brussels Sprouts:** Roast in the oven for 10 minutes until they start to brown. **Season Trout:** Meanwhile, drizzle the trout fillets with the remaining olive oil. Season each fillet with salt and black pepper.
4. **Combine and Roast:** After 10 minutes, push the Brussels sprouts to one side of the baking sheet and place the trout fillets on the other side. Roast for an additional 10 minutes until the trout is cooked through and flakes easily with a fork.
5. **Serve:** Plate the trout fillets alongside the roasted Brussels sprouts. Garnish with fresh herbs if desired, and serve warm.

NUTRITION INFORMATION: (APPROXIMATE VALUES PER SERVING): Calories: 330 | Protein: 28g | Carbohydrates: 10g | Sodium: 180mg | Fats: 20g | Potassium: 590mg | Sugar: 2g | Cholesterol: 55mg

VEGAN BUDDHA BOWL WITH SPICED CHICKPEAS

A balanced and hearty lunch, this Buddha bowl combines roasted, spiced chickpeas with a medley of colorful vegetables, served over quinoa and finished with a tangy tahini dressing.

- **Prep Time:** 15 minutes
- **Cooking Time:** 25 minutes
- **Complexity:** Beginner
- **Servings:** 4
- **Ingredients:** 12

EQUIPMENT NEEDED: Baking sheet, mixing bowl, saucepan, serving bowls, whisk

TAGS: Whole Foods, vegan, Low Glycemic, Heart-Healthy, gluten-free, dairy-free, High-protein, High-fiber, Low Sodium, low-fat, Vitamin A rich, Vitamin C rich

INGREDIENT LIST:

- 1 1/2 cups cooked quinoa (225 g)
- 1 can chickpeas, drained and rinsed (15 oz / 425 g)
- 1 tbsp olive oil (15 mL)
- 1 tsp smoked paprika (5 mL)
- 1 tsp cumin powder (5 mL)
- 1/2 tsp garlic powder (2.5 mL)
- 1/4 tsp salt (1.25 mL)
- 1/4 tsp black pepper (1.25 mL)
- 1 large carrot, shredded
- 1 cucumber, sliced, 1 avocado, diced, 1/4 cup tahini (60 mL)
- Juice of 1 lemon

DIRECTIONS:

1. Preheat the oven to 400°F (200°C). In a mixing bowl, combine chickpeas with olive oil, smoked paprika, cumin powder, garlic powder, salt, and black pepper. Mix well.
2. Spread the seasoned chickpeas on a baking sheet and roast for 20-25 minutes, stirring halfway, until crisp.
3. Meanwhile, cook the quinoa according to package instructions and set aside.
4. In a small bowl, whisk together tahini and lemon juice with a splash of water until smooth.
5. To assemble the Buddha bowls, divide the quinoa evenly into four serving bowls. Top with roasted chickpeas, shredded carrot, sliced cucumber, and diced avocado. Drizzle each bowl with the tahini dressing.

NUTRITION INFORMATION: (APPROXIMATE VALUES PER SERVING): Calories: 330 | Protein: 12 g | Carbohydrates: 44 g | Sodium: 180 mg | Fats: 12 g | Potassium: 700 mg | Sugar: 5 g | Cholesterol: 0 mg

ROASTED VEGETABLE AND FARRO BOWL

This wholesome and satisfying bowl combines roasted seasonal vegetables with nutty farro for a nutrient-rich lunch that's both flavorful and filling.

Prep Time: 15 minutes
Cooking Time: 25 minutes
Complexity: Beginner
Servings: 4
Ingredients: 10

EQUIPMENT NEEDED: Baking sheet, mixing bowl, saucepan, knife, serving bowls
TAGS: Whole Foods, vegetarian, Low Glycemic, Heart-Healthy, High-fiber, Low Sodium, low-fat, Vitamin A rich, Vitamin C rich

INGREDIENT LIST:
- 1 cup farro (170 g)
- 1 medium sweet potato, diced
- 1 zucchini, sliced into rounds
- 1 red bell pepper, diced
- 1 small red onion, quartered
- 2 tbsp olive oil (30 mL)
- 1 tsp ground cumin (5 mL)
- 1/2 tsp smoked paprika (2.5 mL)
- 1/4 tsp salt (1.25 mL)
- 1/4 tsp black pepper (1.25 mL)

DIRECTIONS:
1. Preheat the oven to 425°F (220°C). In a mixing bowl, toss the sweet potato, zucchini, bell pepper, and red onion with olive oil, ground cumin, smoked paprika, salt, and black pepper. Spread the seasoned vegetables on a baking sheet.
2. Roast the vegetables for 20-25 minutes, stirring halfway through, until tender and slightly caramelized.
3. While the vegetables are roasting, cook the farro according to package instructions. Drain any excess water and set aside.
4. To assemble the bowls, divide the farro evenly among four serving bowls. Top with the roasted vegetables and drizzle with additional olive oil if desired.

NUTRITION INFORMATION: (APPROXIMATE VALUES PER SERVING): Calories: 320 | Protein: 7 g | Carbohydrates: 50 g | Sodium: 170 mg | Fats: 9 g | Potassium: 800 mg | Sugar: 7 g | Cholesterol: 0 mg

SPINACH AND MUSHROOM POLENTA STACKS

These savory polenta stacks feature layers of creamy polenta, sautéed mushrooms, and seasoned spinach, providing a hearty yet healthy lunch option.

Prep Time: 20 minutes
Cooking Time: 30 minutes
Complexity: Intermediate
Servings: 4
Ingredients: 10

EQUIPMENT NEEDED: Mixing bowl, saucepan, baking sheet, skillet, spatula, knife
TAGS: Whole Foods, vegetarian, gluten-free, Low Glycemic, Heart-Healthy, High-fiber, Low Sodium, low-fat, Vitamin A rich, Vitamin C rich, Vitamin D rich

INGREDIENT LIST:
- 1 cup polenta (cornmeal) (170 g)
- 4 cups water (1 L)
- 1 tbsp olive oil (15 mL)
- 1 lb mushrooms, sliced (450 g)
- 4 cups fresh spinach (120 g)
- 1 clove garlic, minced
- 1/4 tsp salt (1.25 mL)
- 1/4 tsp black pepper (1.25 mL)
- 1/4 tsp smoked paprika (1.25 mL)
- 1 tsp dried basil (5 mL)

DIRECTIONS:
1. In a saucepan, bring the water to a boil. Slowly whisk in the polenta and reduce to low heat. Stir continuously for 10-15 minutes until thick and creamy. Pour the polenta into a baking sheet and spread evenly. Let it cool and set, then cut into rounds using a cookie cutter or a knife.
2. In a skillet, heat olive oil over medium heat. Add the sliced mushrooms and sauté for 5-7 minutes until browned. Add the minced garlic, salt, black pepper, smoked paprika, and basil. Stir well and cook for another 2-3 minutes.
3. Add the spinach to the skillet and stir until wilted about 2 minutes. Remove from heat.
4. To assemble the stacks, layer a round of polenta on each plate. Top with a portion of the sautéed mushroom and spinach mixture. Repeat the layering with another round of polenta and another spoonful of the vegetable mixture.
5. Serve immediately and enjoy!

NUTRITION INFORMATION: (APPROXIMATE VALUES PER SERVING): Calories: 210 | Protein: 5 g | Carbohydrates: 32 g | Sodium: 180 mg | Fats: 6 g | Potassium: 700 mg | Sugar: 3 g | Cholesterol: 0 mg

BUTTERNUT SQUASH AND CHICKPEA CURRY

A warming, plant-based curry that combines the sweetness of butternut squash with protein-rich chickpeas and aromatic spices. This hearty meal is perfect for a filling, nutrient-rich lunch.

- Prep Time: 15 minutes
- Cooking Time: 30 minutes
- Complexity: Beginner
- Servings: 4
- Ingredients: 10

EQUIPMENT NEEDED: Large saucepan or pot, mixing spoon, knife, cutting board

TAGS: Whole Foods, vegan, Low Glycemic, Heart-Healthy, High-fiber, Low Sodium, low-fat, gluten-free, Vitamin A rich, Vitamin C rich

INGREDIENT LIST:

- 1 tbsp olive oil (15 mL)
- 1 large onion, diced
- 2 cloves garlic, minced
- 1 tbsp curry powder (15 mL)
- 1/2 tsp ground cumin (2.5 mL)
- 1/4 tsp ground cinnamon (1.25 mL)
- 3 cups butternut squash, peeled and diced (450 g)
- 1 can chickpeas, drained and rinsed (15 oz / 425 g)
- 1 can diced tomatoes, no salt added (14 oz / 400 g)
- 1 cup vegetable broth, low sodium (240 mL)

DIRECTIONS:

1. In a large saucepan or pot, heat olive oil over medium heat. Add diced onion and sauté for 5 minutes until softened.
2. Add minced garlic, curry powder, ground cumin, and ground cinnamon to the pot. Stir and cook for 1-2 minutes until aromatic.
3. Add diced butternut squash, chickpeas, diced tomatoes, and vegetable broth to the pot. Stir well to combine.
4. Bring the mixture to a simmer, then reduce the heat to low and cover. Cook for 20-25 minutes or until the squash is tender and the flavors have melded together.
5. Serve hot with your choice of brown rice, quinoa, or greens.

NUTRITION INFORMATION: (APPROXIMATE VALUES PER SERVING): Calories: 280 | Protein: 8 g | Carbohydrates: 45 g | Sodium: 170 mg | Fats: 8 g | Potassium: 900 mg | Sugar: 9 g | Cholesterol: 0 mg

TURMERIC GRILLED CHICKEN AND QUINOA SALAD

This nutritious salad features turmeric-marinated grilled chicken atop a bed of quinoa, mixed greens, and colorful veggies. It's ideal for a healthy, filling lunch.

- Prep Time: 15 minutes
- Cooking Time: 20 minutes
- Complexity: Beginner
- Servings: 4
- Ingredients: 10

EQUIPMENT NEEDED: Mixing bowl, grill pan or outdoor grill, saucepan, salad bowl, tongs, spoon

TAGS: Whole Foods, Heart-Healthy, gluten-free, dairy-free, High-protein, High-fiber, Low Glycemic, low-fat, Low Sodium, Vitamin C rich

INGREDIENT LIST:

- 1 lb boneless, skinless chicken breasts (450 g)
- 1 tsp turmeric powder (5 mL)
- 1 tsp ground cumin (5 mL)
- 1/2 tsp black pepper (2.5 mL)
- 1 tbsp olive oil (15 mL)
- Juice of 1 lemon
- 1 cup quinoa (170 g)
- 4 cups mixed greens (120 g)
- 1 cucumber, sliced
- 1 red bell pepper, diced

DIRECTIONS:

1. In a mixing bowl, combine turmeric powder, cumin, black pepper, olive oil, and lemon juice. Add the chicken breasts to the marinade and coat well. Let sit for 10 minutes.
2. Preheat a grill pan or outdoor grill to medium-high heat. Grill the marinated chicken for 5-6 minutes per side until fully cooked. The internal temperature should reach 165°F (74°C). Let the chicken rest for 5 minutes before slicing.
3. While the chicken is grilling, cook the quinoa according to package instructions. Set aside to cool slightly.
4. In a large salad bowl, combine cooked quinoa, mixed greens, cucumber slices, and diced red bell pepper. Toss lightly to mix.
5. Top the salad with the sliced grilled chicken and serve immediately.

NUTRITION INFORMATION: (APPROXIMATE VALUES PER SERVING): Calories: 320 | Protein: 28 g | Carbohydrates: 35 g | Sodium: 140 mg | Fats: 8 g | Potassium: 900 mg | Sugar: 4 g | Cholesterol: 70 mg

SPECIAL SECTION: LUNCHES ON THE GO

ASPARAGUS AND SHRIMP WITH QUINOA

A light and nutritious breakfast featuring shrimp and asparagus with quinoa, this dish is high in protein, low in fat, and ideal for a fatty liver diet. It's simple to prepare yet offers a hearty combination of flavors.

Prep Time: 10 minutes
Cooking Time: 20 minutes
Complexity: Beginner
Servings: 4
Ingredients: 9

EQUIPMENT NEEDED: Pot, pan, bowl, spoon
TAGS: Whole Foods, Heart-Healthy, Low Glycemic, High-Protein, Low Sodium, Low Fat, Gluten-Free

INGREDIENT LIST:

- 1 cup (190 g) quinoa, rinsed
- 2 cups (480 ml) low-sodium vegetable broth
- 1 tablespoon (15 ml) olive oil
- 1 lb (450 g) asparagus, trimmed and cut into 2-inch pieces
- 1 lb (450 g) shrimp, peeled and deveined
- 2 cloves garlic, minced
- 1 teaspoon (5 ml) lemon zest
- 1 tablespoon (15 ml) lemon juice
- 2 tablespoons (30 ml) fresh parsley, chopped

DIRECTIONS:

1. **Cook Quinoa:** In a pot, bring vegetable broth to a boil. Add rinsed quinoa, reduce heat to low, cover, and simmer for 15 minutes or until all liquid is absorbed. Fluff with a fork and set aside.
2. **Sauté Asparagus:** In a pan, heat olive oil over medium heat. Add asparagus and cook for 4-5 minutes, stirring occasionally, until tender but still crisp.
3. **Cook Shrimp:** Add minced garlic and shrimp to the pan with asparagus. Cook for 3-4 minutes or until shrimp are pink and opaque.
4. **Add Flavor:** Stir in lemon zest, lemon juice, and parsley. Mix well to incorporate.
5. **Combine:** In a large bowl, combine the cooked quinoa with the shrimp and asparagus mixture. Toss gently to combine.
6. **Serve:** Divide the mixture among plates and serve immediately.

NUTRITION INFORMATION: (APPROXIMATE VALUES PER SERVING): Calories: 280 | Protein: 24g | Carbohydrates: 30g | Sodium: 150mg | Fats: 8g | Potassium: 450mg | Sugar: 2g | Cholesterol: 120mg

BALSAMIC GRILLED ZUCCHINI WITH PARMESAN

A simple yet flavorful breakfast recipe that pairs the mild taste of grilled zucchini with the tangy notes of balsamic vinegar and savory Parmesan cheese.

Prep Time: 10 minutes
Cooking Time: 5-7 minutes
Complexity: Beginner
Servings: 4
Ingredients: 6

EQUIPMENT NEEDED: Grill or grill pan, bowl, brush, grater, tongs
TAGS: Low Glycemic, Heart-Healthy, Whole Foods, Low Sodium, Low Fat, Gluten-Free, High Fiber, Vitamin A Rich, Vitamin C Rich

INGREDIENT LIST:

- 4 medium zucchinis, sliced lengthwise
- 2 tablespoons (30 ml) balsamic vinegar, 2 tablespoons (30 ml) extra-virgin olive oil
- 1/2 cup (50 g) freshly grated Parmesan cheese
- Salt and pepper to taste
- Fresh parsley for garnish (optional)

DIRECTIONS:

1. **Prepare Marinade:** In a bowl, whisk together balsamic vinegar and olive oil. Season with salt and pepper.
2. **Marinate Zucchini:** Brush the zucchini slices with the balsamic and olive oil mixture on both sides.
3. **Grill Zucchini:** Preheat the grill or grill pan over medium-high heat. Grill the zucchini slices for 2-3 minutes per side or until grill marks appear and the zucchini becomes tender.
4. **Garnish and Serve:** Transfer the grilled zucchini to a serving plate. Sprinkle with freshly grated Parmesan cheese and garnish with chopped parsley if desired. Serve immediately.

NUTRITION INFORMATION: (APPROXIMATE VALUES PER SERVING): Calories: 120 | Protein: 5g | Carbohydrates: 7g | Sodium: 110mg | Fats: 7g | Potassium: 450mg | Sugar: 4g | Cholesterol: 5mg

EGGPLANT ROLLATINI WITH SPINACH AND RICOTTA

This light yet satisfying lunch option features grilled eggplant slices filled with a savory mixture of spinach and ricotta, then baked in a light tomato sauce.

Prep Time: 20 minutes
Cooking Time: 30 minutes
Complexity: Intermediate
Servings: 4
Ingredients: 9

EQUIPMENT NEEDED: Grill pan or outdoor grill, mixing bowl, baking dish, spoon, measuring cups, knife

TAGS: Whole Foods, vegetarian, gluten-free, Low Glycemic, Heart-Healthy, High-fiber, Low Sodium, low-fat, Vitamin A rich, Vitamin C rich

INGREDIENT LIST:

- 2 large eggplants, sliced lengthwise into 1/4-inch thick strips
- 2 tbsp olive oil (30 mL)
- 1/4 tsp salt (1.25 mL)
- 1/4 tsp black pepper (1.25 mL)
- 1 cup part-skim ricotta cheese (250 g), 1 cup baby spinach, chopped (30 g)
- 1 large egg, lightly beaten, 1/4 cup grated Parmesan cheese (30 g)
- 1 1/2 cups low-sodium tomato sauce (350 mL)

DIRECTIONS:

1. Preheat a grill pan or outdoor grill to medium-high heat. Brush both sides of the eggplant slices with olive oil and season with salt and black pepper. Grill the eggplant slices for 2-3 minutes per side until tender but not falling apart. Set aside. In a mixing bowl, combine ricotta cheese, chopped spinach, beaten egg, and grated Parmesan cheese. Mix well.
2. Preheat the oven to 375°F (190°C). Lay each grilled eggplant slice flat, place a spoonful of the ricotta mixture on one end, and roll up the eggplant. Place the roll, seam-side down, in a baking dish. Repeat with the remaining eggplant slices and filling.
3. Pour the tomato sauce over the rolled eggplant in the baking dish. Cover the dish with foil and bake for 20 minutes. Remove the foil and bake for another 5-10 minutes or until the top is slightly golden.
4. Let cool for 5 minutes before serving.

NUTRITION INFORMATION: (APPROXIMATE VALUES PER SERVING): Calories: 180 | Protein: 10 g | Carbohydrates: 15 g | Sodium: 200 mg | Fats: 8 g | Potassium: 600 mg | Sugar: 6 g | Cholesterol: 25 mg

LEMON GARLIC TILAPIA WITH STEAMED KALE

This heart-healthy lunch combines delicately seasoned tilapia with steamed kale, delivering a flavorful, nutritious meal that's rich in protein and vitamins.

Prep Time: 10 minutes
Cooking Time: 15 minutes
Complexity: Beginner
Servings: 4
Ingredients: 8

EQUIPMENT NEEDED: Baking sheet, mixing bowl, steamer basket, skillet, tongs, knife

TAGS: Whole Foods, gluten-free, dairy-free, High-protein, High-fiber, Low Sodium, low-fat, Low Glycemic, Heart-Healthy, Vitamin C rich, Vitamin A rich

INGREDIENT LIST:

- 4 tilapia fillets (about 1 lb / 450 g)
- 2 tbsp olive oil (30 mL)
- Juice and zest of 1 lemon
- 2 cloves garlic, minced
- 1/4 tsp salt (1.25 mL)
- 1/4 tsp black pepper (1.25 mL)
- 1 bunch kale, stems removed and leaves torn into pieces
- 1/4 tsp smoked paprika (1.25 mL)

DIRECTIONS:

1. Preheat the oven to 375°F (190°C). In a mixing bowl, combine olive oil, lemon juice, lemon zest, minced garlic, salt, black pepper, and smoked paprika. Mix well.
2. Arrange tilapia fillets on a baking sheet lined with parchment paper. Brush the seasoned olive oil mixture over the fillets, coating evenly.
3. Bake the fillets for 12-15 minutes or until they reach an internal temperature of 145°F (63°C) and flake easily with a fork.
4. While the fish is baking, steam the kale in a steamer basket over boiling water for 3-4 minutes or until tender but still vibrant green. Season with salt and a drizzle of lemon juice if desired.
5. Serve each tilapia fillet with a generous portion of steamed kale on the side.

NUTRITION INFORMATION: (APPROXIMATE VALUES PER SERVING): Calories: 220 | Protein: 26 g | Carbohydrates: 8 g | Sodium: 200 mg | Fats: 10 g | Potassium: 700 mg | Sugar: 1 g | Cholesterol: 55 mg

PESTO CHICKEN AND VEGGIE WRAP

This quick and satisfying lunch wrap is made with lean chicken breast, crunchy veggies, and a flavorful pesto. It's perfect for an energizing, heart-healthy meal on the go.

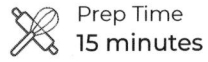

Prep Time: 15 minutes
Cooking Time: 15 minutes
Complexity: Beginner
Servings: 4
Ingredients: 9

EQUIPMENT NEEDED: Skillet, mixing bowl, spoon, knife, serving plates

TAGS: Whole Foods, Low Glycemic, Heart-Healthy, High-protein, High-fiber, Low Sodium, low-fat, Vitamin A rich, Vitamin C rich

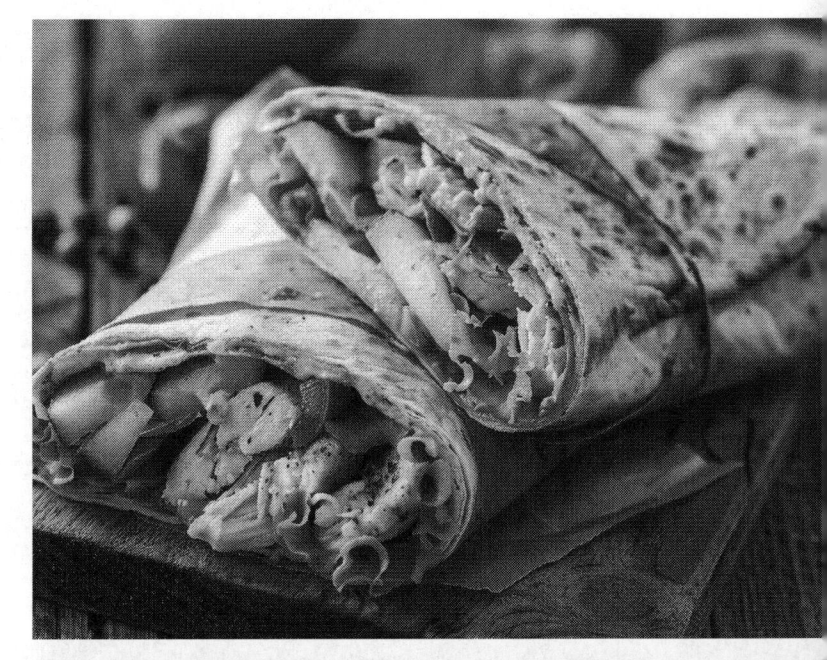

INGREDIENT LIST:

- 1 lb boneless, skinless chicken breasts, cooked and shredded (450 g)
- 4 whole wheat wraps
- 1/4 cup prepared pesto (60 mL)
- 1 cup baby spinach (30 g)
- 1 red bell pepper, thinly sliced
- 1 cucumber, sliced into rounds
- 1 large carrot, shredded
- 1 avocado, sliced
- 1/4 tsp black pepper (1.25 mL)

DIRECTIONS:

1. Warm the whole wheat wraps in a skillet over medium heat for 1-2 minutes per side until pliable. Set aside.
2. In a mixing bowl, toss the shredded chicken with the prepared pesto and black pepper until well combined.
3. To assemble each wrap, layer baby spinach, bell pepper slices, cucumber rounds, shredded carrot, and avocado slices evenly across the middle of the wrap.
4. Add a generous portion of the pesto chicken mixture on top of the veggies.
5. Fold in the sides and roll up the wrap tightly. Slice each wrap in half and serve on a plate.

NUTRITION INFORMATION: (APPROXIMATE VALUES PER SERVING): Calories: 310 | Protein: 26 g | Carbohydrates: 30 g | Sodium: 220 mg | Fats: 10 g | Potassium: 600 mg | Sugar: 5 g | Cholesterol: 50 mg

CHAPTER 5: DELIGHTFUL DINNERS

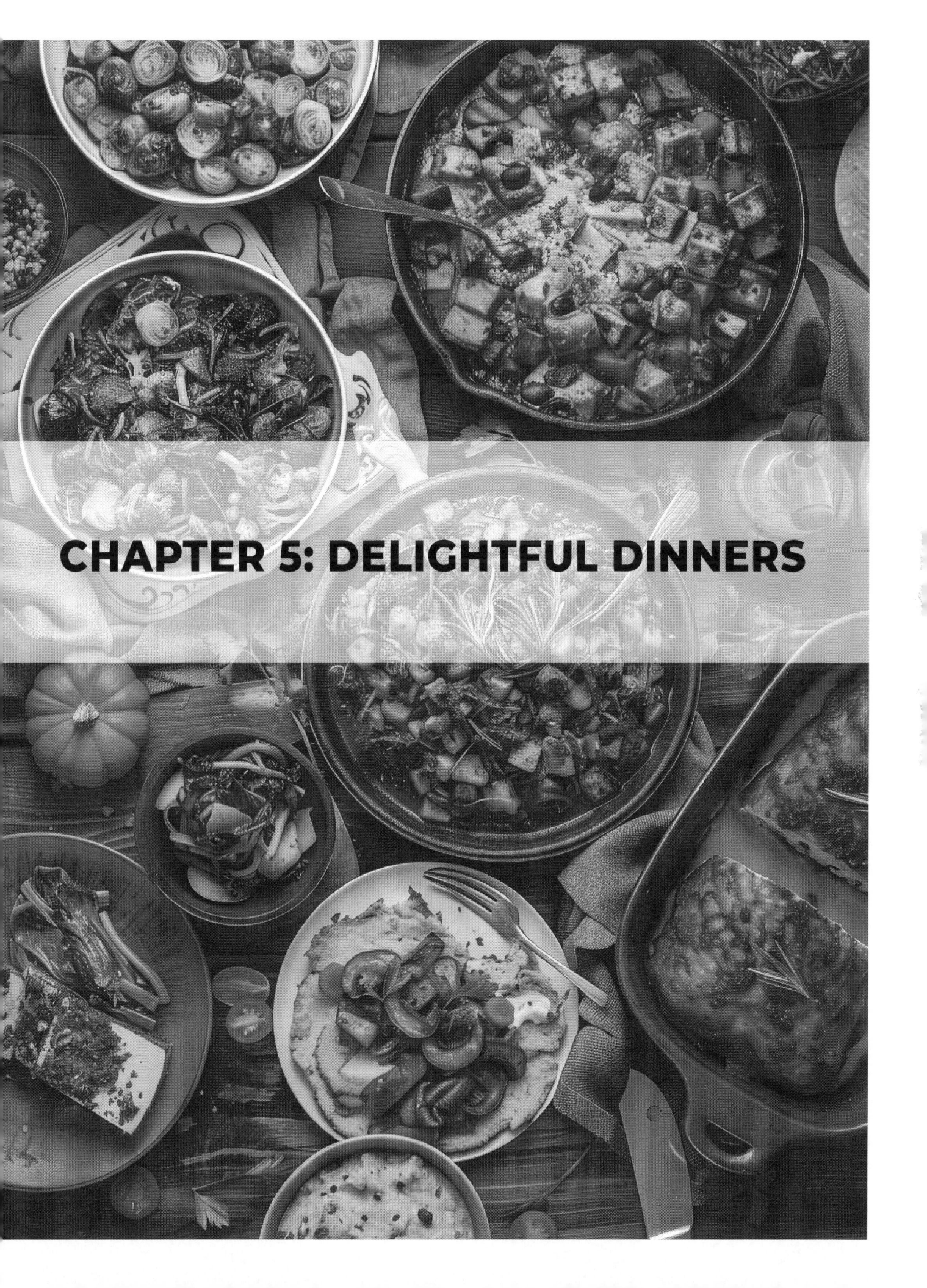

PUMPKIN AND BLACK BEAN CASSEROLE

A cozy and comforting dish, this casserole combines the sweetness of pumpkin with hearty black beans and a savory spice blend, making it a perfect dinner option.

Prep Time: 20 minutes
Cooking Time: 40 minutes
Complexity: Intermediate
Servings: 4
Ingredients: 9

EQUIPMENT NEEDED: Mixing bowl, baking dish, skillet, spoon, knife
TAGS: Whole Foods, vegan, Low Glycemic, Heart-Healthy, High-fiber, Low Sodium, low-fat, Vitamin A rich, Vitamin C rich

INGREDIENT LIST:

- 2 cups diced pumpkin (300 g)
- 1 can black beans, drained and rinsed (15 oz / 425 g)
- 1 large onion, chopped
- 2 cloves garlic, minced
- 1 red bell pepper, diced
- 1 tsp cumin powder (5 mL)
- 1/2 tsp smoked paprika (2.5 mL)
- 1/4 tsp chili powder (1.25 mL)
- 1 cup low-sodium vegetable broth (240 mL)
- Salt and pepper to taste

DIRECTIONS:

1. Preheat the oven to 375°F (190°C). Grease a baking dish with a little olive oil. In a skillet, heat a splash of olive oil over medium heat. Add the onion and garlic, and sauté until translucent, about 5 minutes.
2. Add the red bell pepper, pumpkin, cumin, smoked paprika, and chili powder. Cook for another 5 minutes until the vegetables are slightly softened.
3. Stir in the black beans and vegetable broth. Season with salt and pepper. Bring to a simmer and cook for 5 minutes.
4. Transfer the mixture to the prepared baking dish. Cover with foil and bake in the preheated oven for 30 minutes or until the pumpkin is tender and the flavors are well combined.
5. Remove the foil and bake for an additional 10 minutes to slightly reduce the liquid.
6. Serve hot, garnished with fresh cilantro or parsley if desired.

NUTRITION INFORMATION: (APPROXIMATE VALUES PER SERVING): Calories: 200 | Protein: 8 g | Carbohydrates: 38 g | Sodium: 180 mg | Fats: 2 g | Potassium: 600 mg | Sugar: 5 g | Cholesterol: 0 mg

CREAMY BROCCOLI AND SPINACH SOUP

This deliciously creamy soup combines nutrient-rich broccoli and spinach in a comforting dish, making it a perfect dinner option for promoting liver health and overall wellness.

Prep Time: 10 minutes
Cooking Time: 20 minutes
Complexity: Beginner
Servings: 4
Ingredients: 8

EQUIPMENT NEEDED: Large pot, blender or immersion blender, knife, cutting board, measuring cups
TAGS: Whole Foods, vegan, Low Glycemic, Heart-Healthy, High-fiber, Low Sodium, low-fat, gluten-free, dairy-free, Vitamin A rich, Vitamin C rich

INGREDIENT LIST:

- 1 tbsp olive oil (15 mL)
- 1 onion, chopped
- 2 cloves garlic, minced
- 4 cups broccoli florets (about 1 large head)
- 3 cups fresh spinach (90 g)
- 4 cups low-sodium vegetable broth (1 L)
- 1/2 cup unsweetened almond milk (120 mL)
- Salt and pepper to taste

DIRECTIONS:

1. Heat olive oil in a large pot over medium heat. Add the chopped onion and garlic and sauté until the onion is translucent, about 5 minutes.
2. Add the broccoli florets to the pot and stir to combine. Cook for another 5 minutes, just until the broccoli starts to soften.
3. Pour in the vegetable broth and bring the mixture to a boil. Reduce heat and simmer for 10 minutes or until the broccoli is completely tender. Add the fresh spinach and cook for an additional 2-3 minutes, until the spinach has wilted.
4. Remove the pot from heat. Using a blender or an immersion blender, puree the soup until it is completely smooth. Stir in the almond milk and season with salt and pepper to taste. Reheat gently if necessary.
5. Serve hot, garnished with a drizzle of olive oil or a sprinkle of nutritional yeast if desired.

NUTRITION INFORMATION: (APPROXIMATE VALUES PER SERVING): Calories: 110 | Protein: 5 g | Carbohydrates: 15 g | Sodium: 150 mg | Fats: 4 g | Potassium: 480 mg | Sugar: 4 g | Cholesterol: 0 mg

SAUTÉED BRUSSELS SPROUTS WITH CRISPY TOFU

This dish combines the heartiness of crispy tofu with the earthy flavors of Brussels sprouts, creating a nutrient-rich, satisfying dinner that supports liver health and overall wellness.

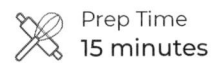

- **Prep Time:** 15 minutes
- **Cooking Time:** 25 minutes
- **Complexity:** Intermediate
- **Servings:** 4
- **Ingredients:** 8

EQUIPMENT NEEDED: Large skillet, baking sheet, mixing bowl, knife, tongs

TAGS: Whole Foods, vegan, Low Glycemic, Heart-Healthy, gluten-free, dairy-free, High-protein, High-fiber, Low Sodium, low-fat, Vitamin C rich

INGREDIENT LIST:

- 1 lb Brussels sprouts, halved (450 g)
- 14 oz extra-firm tofu, pressed and cubed (400 g)
- 2 tbsp olive oil (30 mL)
- 1 tsp garlic powder (5 mL)
- 1/2 tsp smoked paprika (2.5 mL)
- Salt and pepper to taste
- 1 tbsp soy sauce, low sodium (15 mL)
- 1 tbsp balsamic vinegar (15 mL)

DIRECTIONS:

1. Preheat your oven to 400°F (200°C). Toss the cubed tofu with 1 tablespoon of olive oil, soy sauce, garlic powder, and smoked paprika. Spread on a baking sheet and bake for 20-25 minutes until crispy, turning halfway through cooking.
2. While the tofu is baking, heat the remaining olive oil in a large skillet over medium heat. Add the halved Brussels sprouts, salt, and pepper. Sauté for about 10-12 minutes, stirring occasionally, until the sprouts are tender and caramelized on the edges.
3. In the last minute of cooking the Brussels sprouts, drizzle balsamic vinegar over them and stir to coat evenly.
4. Combine the crispy tofu and sautéed Brussels sprouts in a serving dish, gently tossing to mix.
5. Serve warm, optionally garnished with fresh herbs like parsley or thyme for added flavor.

NUTRITION INFORMATION: (APPROXIMATE VALUES PER SERVING): Calories: 250 | Protein: 15 g | Carbohydrates: 18 g | Sodium: 200 mg | Fats: 15 g | Potassium: 700 mg | Sugar: 4 g | Cholesterol: 0 mg

STUFFED PORTOBELLO MUSHROOMS WITH SPINACH AND PINE NUTS

This delicious and nutritious dinner features large Portobello mushrooms stuffed with a flavorful mixture of spinach and pine nuts, making it perfect for a satisfying, low-carb evening meal.

- **Prep Time:** 15 minutes
- **Cooking Time:** 20 minutes
- **Complexity:** Beginner
- **Servings:** 4
- **Ingredients:** 8

EQUIPMENT NEEDED: Baking sheet, skillet, mixing bowl, spoon, knife

TAGS: Whole Foods, vegetarian, gluten-free, Low Glycemic, Heart-Healthy, High-fiber, Low Sodium, low-fat, Vitamin A rich, Vitamin C rich, Vitamin D rich

INGREDIENT LIST:

- 4 large Portobello mushroom caps, stems, and gills removed
- 1 tbsp olive oil (15 mL)
- 2 cups fresh spinach, chopped (60 g)
- 1/4 cup pine nuts (30 g)
- 2 cloves garlic, minced
- 1/2 tsp salt (2.5 mL)
- 1/4 tsp black pepper (1.25 mL)
- 1/4 cup grated Parmesan cheese, optional (for non-vegan option) (30 g)

DIRECTIONS:

1. Preheat the oven to 375°F (190°C). Line a baking sheet with parchment paper. Heat olive oil in a skillet over medium heat. Add garlic and sauté for 1 minute until fragrant.
2. Add the spinach to the skillet and cook until wilted, about 3-4 minutes. Stir in the pine nuts, salt, and pepper, and cook for an additional 2 minutes.
3. Place the Portobello mushrooms on the prepared baking sheet, gill-side up. Divide the spinach and pine nut mixture evenly among the mushrooms, packing it into the caps.
4. If using, sprinkle grated Parmesan cheese over the top of each stuffed mushroom.
5. Bake in the preheated oven for 15-20 minutes or until the mushrooms are tender and the filling is heated through. Serve warm, garnished with additional pine nuts or fresh herbs if desired.

NUTRITION INFORMATION: (APPROXIMATE VALUES PER SERVING): Calories: 150 | Protein: 5 g | Carbohydrates: 10 g | Sodium: 300 mg | Fats: 10 g | Potassium: 400 mg | Sugar: 3 g | Cholesterol: 4 mg

VEGETABLE AND TOFU PAD THAI

This light and flavorful Pad Thai substitutes traditional noodles with strips of vegetables for a nutrient-rich, low glycemic meal that's perfect for supporting liver health.

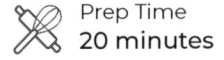

- **Prep Time:** 20 minutes
- **Cooking Time:** 15 minutes
- **Complexity:** Intermediate
- **Servings:** 4
- **Ingredients:** 10

EQUIPMENT NEEDED: Large skillet or wok, knife, cutting board, mixing bowl

TAGS: Whole Foods, vegan, Low Glycemic, Heart-Healthy, gluten-free, dairy-free, High-protein, High-fiber, Low Sodium, low-fat, Vitamin C rich

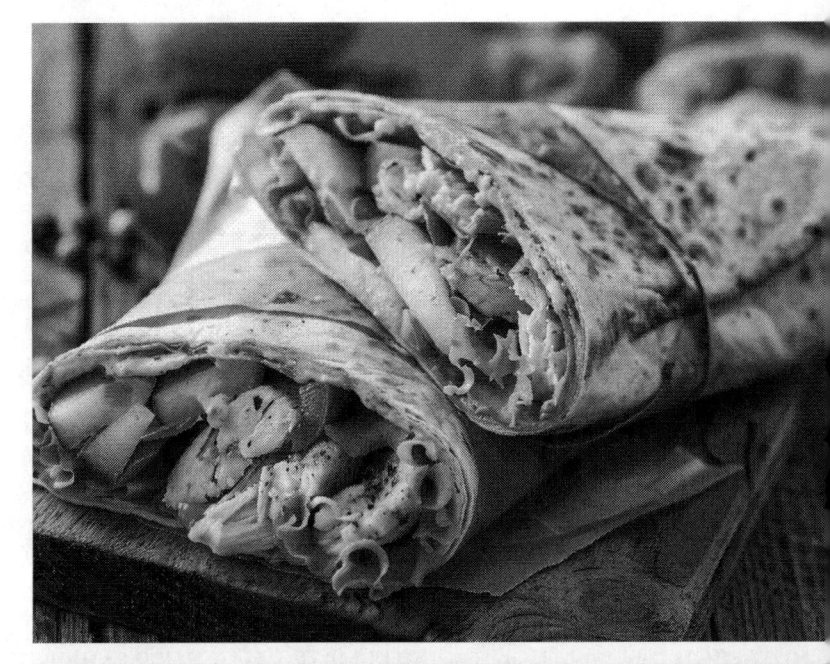

INGREDIENT LIST:

- 1 block (14 oz) firm tofu, pressed and cut into cubes (400 g)
- 2 large carrots, peeled and spiralized or julienned
- 2 zucchinis, spiralized or julienned
- 1 red bell pepper, thinly sliced
- 1 cup bean sprouts (100 g)
- 2 cloves garlic, minced
- 1 tbsp fresh ginger, grated (15 mL)
- 2 tbsp low-sodium soy sauce or tamari (30 mL)
- 1 tbsp lime juice (15 mL)
- 2 tbsp chopped peanuts (for garnish)
- Fresh cilantro (for garnish)

DIRECTIONS:

1. Heat a tablespoon of olive oil in a large skillet or wok over medium-high heat. Add the tofu cubes and fry until golden and crispy, about 5-7 minutes. Remove from the skillet and set aside.
2. In the same skillet, add another tablespoon of olive oil, then sauté garlic and ginger for 1 minute until fragrant.
3. Add the spiralized carrots, zucchini, and sliced bell pepper to the skillet. Stir-fry for about 5 minutes until the vegetables are just tender.
4. Return the tofu to the skillet. Add the soy sauce (or tamari) and lime juice, tossing everything to combine and heat through.
5. Stir in the bean sprouts and cook for an additional minute.
6. Serve hot, garnished with chopped peanuts and fresh cilantro.

NUTRITION INFORMATION: (APPROXIMATE VALUES PER SERVING): Calories: 250 | Protein: 12 g | Carbohydrates: 18 g | Sodium: 200 mg | Fats: 12 g | Potassium: 600 mg | Sugar: 6 g | Cholesterol: 0 mg

CITRUS ROASTED TURKEY BREAST

A delightful dish featuring turkey breast marinated in a blend of citrus juices and herbs, roasted to perfection. This meal is a great source of lean protein and is enriched with the refreshing zest of citrus, making it an ideal choice for a nutritious dinner.

Prep Time: 15 minutes | **Cooking Time:** 45 minutes | **Complexity:** Intermediate | **Servings:** 4 | **Ingredients:** 9

EQUIPMENT NEEDED: Roasting pan, zester, small bowl, whisk, kitchen brush, aluminum foil, meat thermometer

TAGS: Whole Foods, Heart-Healthy, High-protein, Low Sodium, low-fat, gluten-free, High-fiber, Vitamin C rich, Low Glycemic

INGREDIENT LIST:

- 1 1/2 lbs turkey breast, boneless and skinless (about 680 g)
- Juice of 1 orange (about 1/4 cup or 60 mL)
- Juice of 1 lemon (about 2 tbsp or 30 mL)
- 2 tbsp olive oil (30 mL)
- 2 cloves garlic, minced
- 1 tsp fresh thyme, chopped (5 mL)
- 1 tsp fresh rosemary, chopped (5 mL)
- Salt and pepper to taste
- Orange and lemon zest for garnish

DIRECTIONS:

1. In a small bowl, whisk together the orange juice, lemon juice, olive oil, garlic, thyme, rosemary, salt, and pepper.
2. Place the turkey breast in a shallow dish and pour the marinade over it. Cover and refrigerate for at least 2 hours, preferably overnight, to allow the flavors to infuse.
3. Preheat the oven to 375°F (190°C). Place the marinated turkey breast in a roasting pan. Brush some of the marinade over the top.
4. Roast in the preheated oven for approximately 45 minutes, or until the turkey reaches an internal temperature of 165°F (74°C), basting occasionally with the marinade.
5. Once cooked, cover the turkey with aluminum foil and let it rest for 10 minutes before slicing. This helps retain the juices and ensure moistness.
6. Serve the sliced turkey garnished with orange and lemon zest, alongside a side of steamed vegetables or a salad.

NUTRITION INFORMATION: (APPROXIMATE VALUES PER SERVING): Calories: 240 | Protein: 35 g | Carbohydrates: 4 g | Sodium: 75 mg | Fats: 10 g | Potassium: 450 mg | Sugar: 3 g | Cholesterol: 85 mg

ROASTED CAULIFLOWER AND CHICKPEA TACOS

Enjoy a vibrant and healthful dinner with these tacos, featuring spiced roasted cauliflower and chickpeas wrapped in gluten-free corn tortillas. This meal is packed with fiber, protein, and flavorful herbs, perfect for a satisfying yet healthy dinner option.

Prep Time: 15 minutes | **Cooking Time:** 25 minutes | **Complexity:** Beginner | **Servings:** 4 | **Ingredients:** 10

EQUIPMENT NEEDED: Baking sheet, large bowl, skillet, measuring spoons, knife

TAGS: Whole Foods, vegan, Low Glycemic, Heart-Healthy, gluten-free, dairy-free, High-protein, High-fiber, Low Sodium, low-fat, Vitamin C rich

INGREDIENT LIST:

- 1 head cauliflower, cut into small florets, 1 can (15 oz) chickpeas, drained and rinsed
- 1 tbsp olive oil (15 mL)
- 1 tsp chili powder (5 mL)
- 1/2 tsp ground cumin (2.5 mL)
- 1/4 tsp garlic powder (1.25 mL)
- Salt and pepper to taste
- 8 small gluten-free corn tortillas
- 1 avocado, sliced
- 1/4 cup fresh cilantro, chopped (15 g)

DIRECTIONS:

1. Preheat the oven to 400°F (200°C). In a large bowl, toss the cauliflower florets and chickpeas with olive oil, chili powder, cumin, garlic powder, salt, and pepper until well coated.
2. Spread the cauliflower and chickpeas in a single layer on a baking sheet. Roast in the oven for 25 minutes, stirring halfway through, until the cauliflower is tender and slightly crispy.
3. Heat the corn tortillas in a skillet over medium heat for about 30 seconds on each side or until warm and pliable.
4. To assemble the tacos, distribute the roasted cauliflower and chickpeas evenly among the warmed tortillas. Top each taco with avocado slices and a sprinkle of fresh cilantro.
5. Serve immediately, accompanied by lime wedges if desired.

NUTRITION INFORMATION: (APPROXIMATE VALUES PER SERVING): Calories: 350 | Protein: 12 g | Carbohydrates: 45 g | Sodium: 300 mg | Fats: 15 g | Potassium: 600 mg | Sugar: 7 g | Cholesterol: 0 mg

STIR-FRIED KALE AND QUINOA

This stir-fry pairs the robust flavors of kale with the nutty essence of quinoa, creating a fiber-rich, protein-packed dish that's both satisfying and beneficial for maintaining a healthy liver.

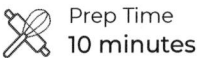

Prep Time: 10 minutes
Cooking Time: 20 minutes
Complexity: Beginner
Servings: 4
Ingredients: 8

EQUIPMENT NEEDED: Large skillet or wok, saucepan, spatula, knife, cutting board
TAGS: Whole Foods, vegan, Low Glycemic, Heart-Healthy, gluten-free, dairy-free, High-protein, High-fiber, Low Sodium, low-fat, Vitamin A rich, Vitamin C rich

INGREDIENT LIST:

- 1 cup quinoa, rinsed (190 g)
- 2 cups water (480 mL)
- 2 tbsp olive oil (30 mL)
- 4 cups chopped kale (about 200 g)
- 1 red bell pepper, thinly sliced
- 2 cloves garlic, minced
- 2 tbsp low sodium soy sauce or tamari (30 mL)
- 1 tbsp sesame seeds (optional, for garnish)

DIRECTIONS:

1. In a saucepan, bring 2 cups of water to a boil. Add quinoa, reduce heat to low, cover, and simmer for 15 minutes or until all water is absorbed. Remove from heat and let sit, covered, for 5 minutes. Fluff with a fork.
2. While the quinoa is cooking, heat olive oil in a large skillet or wok over medium-high heat. Add garlic and sauté for 1 minute until fragrant.
3. Add the chopped kale and red bell pepper to the skillet. Stir-fry for about 5-7 minutes, until the kale is wilted and the peppers are tender but still crisp.
4. Stir in the cooked quinoa and soy sauce. Mix well to combine all ingredients and cook for an additional 2-3 minutes to allow flavors to meld.
5. Serve hot, garnished with sesame seeds if using.

NUTRITION INFORMATION: (APPROXIMATE VALUES PER SERVING): Calories: 250 | Protein: 9 g | Carbohydrates: 35 g | Sodium: 200 mg | Fats: 10 g | Potassium: 600 mg | Sugar: 2 g | Cholesterol: 0 mg

BLACKENED CATFISH WITH COLLARD GREENS

Savor the bold flavors of this southern-inspired dish featuring blackened catfish paired with nutrient-rich collard greens. A perfect combination to support liver health while enjoying a comforting meal.

Prep Time: 15 minutes
Cooking Time: 20 minutes
Complexity: Beginner
Servings: 4
Ingredients: 9

EQUIPMENT NEEDED: Skillet, large pot, stirring spoon, measuring spoons, knife
TAGS: Whole Foods, Heart-Healthy, High-protein, High-fiber, Low Sodium, low-fat, Vitamin A rich, Vitamin C rich, Vitamin D rich

INGREDIENT LIST:

- 4 catfish fillets (about 6 oz each)
- 1 tbsp paprika (15 mL)
- 1 tsp garlic powder (5 mL)
- 1 tsp onion powder (5 mL)
- 1/2 tsp cayenne pepper (2.5 mL)
- 1/2 tsp black pepper (2.5 mL)
- 1 tbsp olive oil (15 mL)
- 1 lb collard greens, stems removed and leaves chopped (450 g)
- 3 cups low-sodium chicken or vegetable broth (720 mL)

DIRECTIONS:

1. Combine paprika, garlic powder, onion powder, cayenne pepper, and black pepper in a small bowl. Rub this spice mix evenly over both sides of the catfish fillets.
2. Heat olive oil in a skillet over medium-high heat. Once hot, add the catfish fillets and cook for about 3-4 minutes on each side or until the outside is crispy and the fish flakes easily with a fork.
3. In a large pot, bring the low-sodium broth to a boil. Add the chopped collard greens, reduce heat to low, and simmer for about 15-20 minutes until the greens are tender.
4. Serve the blackened catfish with a side of braised collard greens.

NUTRITION INFORMATION: (APPROXIMATE VALUES PER SERVING): Calories: 320 | Protein: 35 g | Carbohydrates: 10 g | Sodium: 250 mg | Fats: 15 g | Potassium: 840 mg | Sugar: 2 g | Cholesterol: 85 mg

COD IN PARSLEY CREAM SAUCE

Delight in this tender, flaky cod draped in a light, creamy parsley sauce, offering a nourishing yet indulgent experience. Perfect for a balanced meal that supports liver health without sacrificing taste.

- **Prep Time:** 10 minutes
- **Cooking Time:** 20 minutes
- **Complexity:** Beginner
- **Servings:** 4
- **Ingredients:** 8

EQUIPMENT NEEDED: Skillet, small saucepan, whisk, knife, cutting board

TAGS: Whole Foods, Heart-Healthy, High-protein, Low Sodium, low-fat, Vitamin C rich, Low Glycemic, gluten-free, Sugar-Free

INGREDIENT LIST:

- 4 cod fillets (6 oz each)
- 1 tbsp olive oil (15 mL)
- Salt and pepper to taste
- 1 cup low-fat milk (240 mL)
- 1 tbsp gluten-free flour (15 mL)
- 1/2 cup fresh parsley, finely chopped (30 g)
- 1 clove garlic, minced
- Juice of 1 lemon (about 2 tbsp or 30 mL)

DIRECTIONS:

1. Heat olive oil in a skillet over medium heat. Season the cod fillets with salt and pepper and place them in the skillet. Cook for 4-5 minutes on each side or until the fish flakes easily with a fork. Remove from skillet and set aside.
2. In the same skillet, reduce heat to low. Add garlic and sauté for 1 minute until fragrant. Sprinkle gluten-free flour over the garlic and stir for another minute to cook the flour.
3. Gradually whisk in the low-fat milk, stirring continuously until the mixture thickens into a sauce, about 3-5 minutes. Stir in the chopped parsley and lemon juice, and season with salt and pepper to taste. Cook for an additional 2 minutes to let the flavors meld.
4. Return the cooked cod fillets to the skillet, spooning the sauce over them to reheat the fish for about 2 minutes.
5. Serve the cod fillets immediately, topped with the creamy parsley sauce.

NUTRITION INFORMATION: (APPROXIMATE VALUES PER SERVING): Calories: 200 | Protein: 27 g | Carbohydrates: 5 g | Sodium: 125 mg | Fats: 8 g | Potassium: 620 mg | Sugar: 2 g | Cholesterol: 60 mg

ROASTED BEET AND FETA SALAD

This Roasted Beet and Feta Salad is a colorful, nutrient-rich dish perfect for a healthy dinner. It's loaded with fiber and good fats, making it ideal for a fatty liver diet.

- **Prep Time:** 20 minutes
- **Cooking Time:** 40 minutes
- **Complexity:** Beginner
- **Servings:** 4
- **Ingredients:** 8

EQUIPMENT NEEDED: Oven, roasting tray, mixing bowl, knife, cutting board

TAGS: Whole Foods, vegetarian, Low Glycemic, Heart-Healthy, High-fiber, Low Sodium, Vitamin C rich

INGREDIENT LIST:

- 4 medium beets (about 1 lb or 450g), peeled and diced
- 1 tablespoon olive oil (15 ml)
- 1/4 teaspoon salt (1.25 ml)
- 1/4 teaspoon black pepper (1.25 ml)
- 4 cups arugula (about 120g)
- 1/2 cup crumbled feta cheese (about 75g)
- 1/4 cup chopped walnuts (30g)
- 2 tablespoons balsamic vinegar (30 ml)

DIRECTIONS:

1. Preheat your oven to 400°F (200°C). Toss the diced beets with olive oil, salt, and pepper. Spread them out on a roasting tray.
2. Roast the beets in the preheated oven for about 40 minutes or until tender and slightly caramelized, stirring halfway through.
3. While the beets are roasting, place arugula in a large salad bowl.
4. Once the beets are done, let them cool slightly, then add them to the arugula. Add the crumbled feta cheese and chopped walnuts to the bowl.
5. Drizzle the balsamic vinegar over the salad and toss everything together until well-mixed.
6. Serve immediately or chill in the refrigerator for an hour before serving if preferred cold.

NUTRITION INFORMATION: (APPROXIMATE VALUES PER SERVING): Carbohydrates: 18g | Sodium: 300mg | Fats: 10g | Potassium: 400mg | Sugar: 9g | Cholesterol: 15mg

GRILLED SWORDFISH WITH MEDITERRANEAN SALAD

This savory grilled swordfish paired with a refreshing Mediterranean salad is a hearty, healthful dish packed with lean protein and vibrant vegetables. Ideal for a delicious dinner that aligns with a fatty liver-friendly diet.

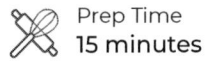

Prep Time: 15 minutes
Cooking Time: 10 minutes
Complexity: Beginner
Servings: 4
Ingredients: 11

EQUIPMENT NEEDED: grill or grill pan, mixing bowl, knife, cutting board

TAGS: High-protein, Low Sodium, Low Glycemic, Heart-Healthy, Whole Foods, High-fiber, low-fat, Vitamin C rich, Sugar-Free

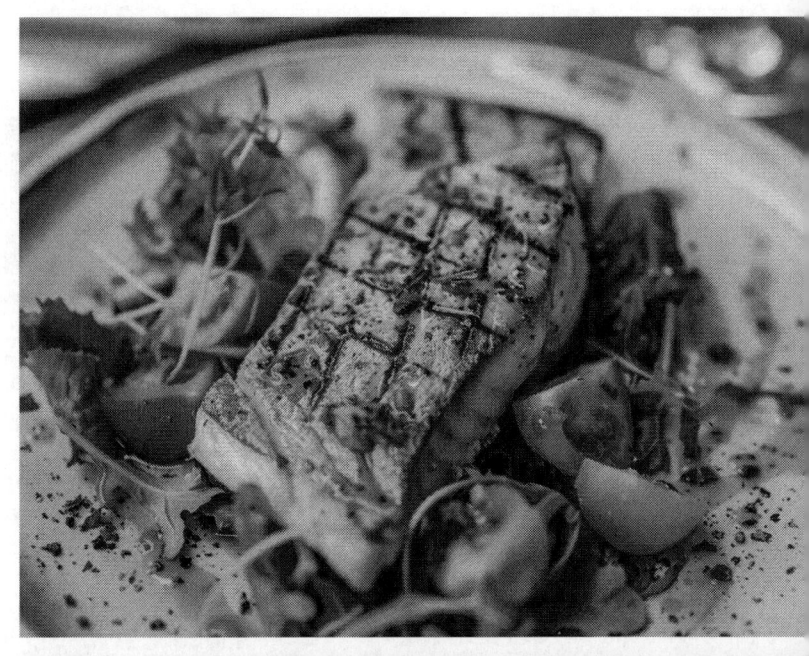

INGREDIENT LIST:

- 4 swordfish steaks (6 oz each)
- 2 tbsp olive oil (30 mL)
- Juice of 1 lemon (about 2 tbsp or 30 mL)
- 2 cloves garlic, minced
- Salt and pepper to taste
- 1 cup cherry tomatoes, halved (150 g)
- 1 cucumber, diced (200 g)
- 1/2 red onion, thinly sliced
- 1/4 cup pitted Kalamata olives, halved (about 30 g)
- 1/4 cup crumbled feta cheese, low-fat (about 30 g)
- 1/4 cup fresh parsley, chopped (about 15 g)

DIRECTIONS:

1. Preheat the grill to medium-high heat. In a small bowl, whisk together olive oil, lemon juice, garlic, salt, and pepper. Brush the swordfish steaks with half of the marinade.
2. Grill the swordfish steaks for about 4-5 minutes on each side or until the fish is cooked through and has grill marks.
3. In a large mixing bowl, combine cherry tomatoes, cucumber, red onion, Kalamata olives, and parsley. Drizzle the remaining marinade over the salad and toss to coat evenly.
4. Divide the salad among plates and top each with a grilled swordfish steak. Sprinkle with feta cheese before serving.

NUTRITION INFORMATION: (APPROXIMATE VALUES PER SERVING): Calories: 350 | Protein: 35 g | Carbohydrates: 9 g | Sodium: 320 mg | Fats: 19 g | Potassium: 850 mg | Sugar: 4 g | Cholesterol: 60 mg

BUTTERNUT SQUASH AND SAGE RISOTTO

This Butternut Squash and Sage Risotto offers a comforting, creamy texture with the sweet richness of squash paired with aromatic sage, perfect for a wholesome dinner.

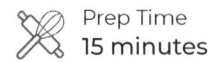

- **Prep Time:** 15 minutes
- **Cooking Time:** 35 minutes
- **Complexity:** Intermediate
- **Servings:** 4
- **Ingredients:** 9

EQUIPMENT NEEDED: Saucepan, wooden spoon, knife, cutting board

TAGS: Whole Foods, vegetarian, Low Glycemic, Heart-Healthy, High-fiber, Low Sodium, Vitamin A rich

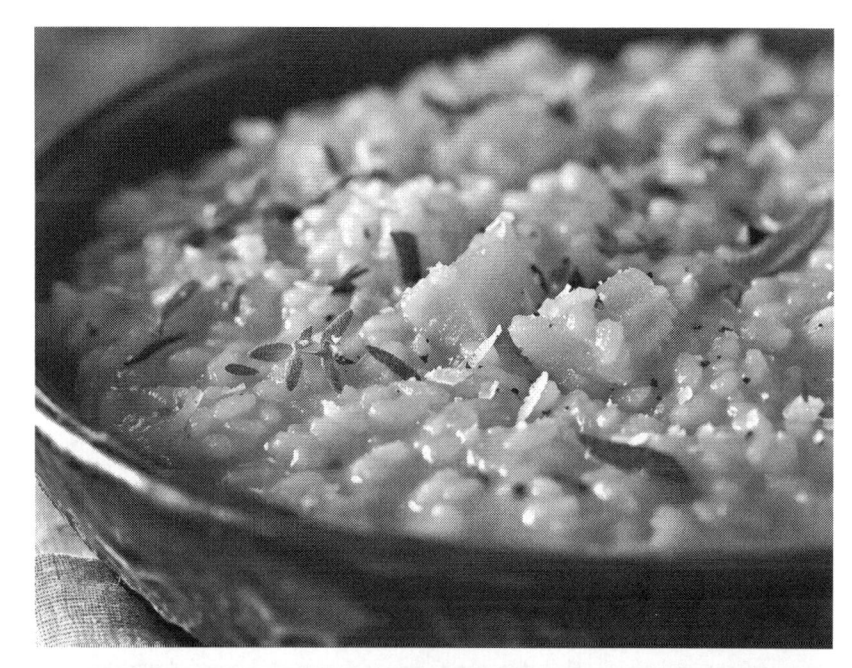

INGREDIENT LIST:

- 1 medium butternut squash (about 2 lbs or 900g), peeled, seeded, and cubed
- 1 tablespoon olive oil (15 ml)
- 1 small onion, finely chopped
- 2 cloves garlic, minced
- 1 cup arborio rice (190g)
- 4 cups low-sodium vegetable broth (950 ml), kept warm
- 1/2 cup dry white wine (120 ml)
- 1/4 cup grated Parmesan cheese (about 30g)
- 2 tablespoons fresh sage, chopped (30 ml)

DIRECTIONS:

1. Preheat your oven to 400°F (200°C). Toss cubed butternut squash with olive oil and spread on a baking sheet. Roast for 25 minutes or until tender.
2. In a large saucepan, heat a splash of olive oil over medium heat. Add onion and garlic, cooking until soft, about 5 minutes.
3. Stir in the arborio rice, coating it with the oil until slightly translucent, about 2 minutes. Add the white wine to the rice mixture, stirring until fully absorbed.
4. Begin adding the warm vegetable broth one cup at a time, stirring constantly and allowing each addition to be absorbed before adding the next. This should take about 20 minutes.
5. Once the rice is tender and creamy, stir in the roasted butternut squash, fresh sage, and Parmesan cheese. Mix until well combined and heated through. Adjust seasoning with salt and pepper to taste, and serve immediately.

NUTRITION INFORMATION: (APPROXIMATE VALUES PER SERVING): Carbohydrates: 58g | Sodium: 240mg | Fats: 8g | Potassium: 530mg | Sugar: 4g | Cholesterol: 5mg

MOROCCAN SPICED FISH WITH COUSCOUS

This flavorful Moroccan Spiced Fish with Couscous is a delightful blend of spices and textures, offering a heart-healthy and high protein meal perfect for supporting liver health.

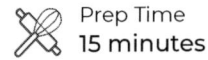

- **Prep Time:** 15 minutes
- **Cooking Time:** 20 minutes
- **Complexity:** Intermediate
- **Servings:** 4
- **Ingredients:** 10

EQUIPMENT NEEDED: Pan, bowl, cutting board, knife, spoon
TAGS: Whole Foods, Heart-Healthy, High-protein, Low Sodium, Low Glycemic

INGREDIENT LIST:

- 4 fillets of white fish such as cod or tilapia (about 6 oz or 170g each)
- 1 tablespoon olive oil (15 ml)
- 1 teaspoon ground cumin (5 ml)
- 1 teaspoon ground coriander (5 ml)
- 1/2 teaspoon ground cinnamon (2.5 ml), 1 cup whole wheat couscous (180g)
- 2 cups low-sodium vegetable broth (475 ml), 1/2 cup diced red bell pepper (about 75g)
- 1/4 cup raisins (about 40g)
- 1/4 cup chopped fresh cilantro (15g) for garnish

DIRECTIONS:

1. Mix cumin, coriander, and cinnamon in a small bowl. Rub the spice mixture over the fish fillets.
2. Heat olive oil in a pan over medium heat. Add the spiced fish fillets and cook for about 4-5 minutes on each side, or until the fish is cooked through and flakes easily with a fork.
3. While the fish is cooking, bring the vegetable broth to a boil in a saucepan. Stir in the couscous, red bell pepper, and raisins. Remove from heat, cover, and let stand for 5 minutes or until the liquid is absorbed.
4. Fluff the couscous with a fork and divide among plates.
5. Place a cooked fish fillet on top of each serving of couscous. Garnish with chopped cilantro.
6. Serve immediately.

NUTRITION INFORMATION: (APPROXIMATE VALUES PER SERVING): Carbohydrates: 45g | Sodium: 180mg | Fats: 7g | Potassium: 650mg | Sugar: 5g | Cholesterol: 55mg

BAKED HAKE WITH SWEET POTATO WEDGES

This dish pairs the light, flaky texture of hake with the natural sweetness of baked sweet potato wedges, providing a nutritious, balanced meal that supports liver health.

- **Prep Time:** 15 minutes
- **Cooking Time:** 25 minutes
- **Complexity:** Beginner
- **Servings:** 4
- **Ingredients:** 7

EQUIPMENT NEEDED: Baking sheet, bowl, knife, cutting board
TAGS: Whole Foods, Heart-Healthy, High-protein, High-fiber, Low Sodium, gluten-free

INGREDIENT LIST:

- 4 hake fillets (about 6 oz or 170g each)
- 2 large sweet potatoes, cut into wedges
- 2 tablespoons olive oil (30 ml)
- 1 teaspoon smoked paprika (5 ml)
- 1/2 teaspoon garlic powder (2.5 ml)
- Fresh parsley, chopped for garnish
- Salt and pepper to taste

DIRECTIONS:

1. Preheat the oven to 400°F (200°C). Line a baking sheet with parchment paper.
2. Toss sweet potato wedges with 1 tablespoon of olive oil, smoked paprika, garlic powder, and a pinch of salt and pepper. Arrange on one half of the baking sheet.
3. Place the hake fillets on the other half of the baking sheet. Brush with the remaining tablespoon of olive oil and season with salt and pepper.
4. Bake in the preheated oven for 20-25 minutes, or until the fish flakes easily with a fork and the sweet potatoes are tender and golden.
5. Serve the baked hake and sweet potato wedges garnished with fresh parsley.

NUTRITION INFORMATION: (APPROXIMATE VALUES PER SERVING): Carbohydrates: 28g | Sodium: 70mg | Fats: 12g | Potassium: 800mg | Sugar: 5g | Cholesterol: 55mg

SPAGHETTI SQUASH PAD THAI

This Spaghetti Squash Pad Thai offers a light and flavorful alternative to traditional Pad Thai, using spaghetti squash instead of noodles for a low-carb, high-fiber meal that supports liver health.

Prep Time: 20 minutes
Cooking Time: 45 minutes
Complexity: Intermediate
Servings: 4
Ingredients: 12

EQUIPMENT NEEDED: Oven, large skillet, fork, knife, cutting board, mixing bowl

TAGS: Whole Foods, vegetarian, gluten-free, Low Glycemic, Heart-Healthy, High-fiber, Low Sodium

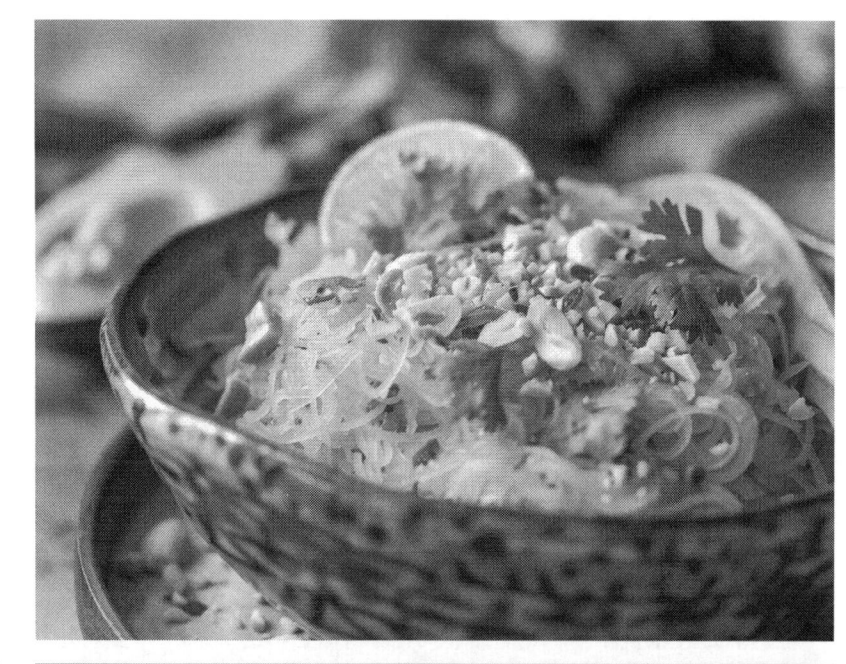

INGREDIENT LIST:

- 1 medium spaghetti squash (about 2 lbs or 900g)
- 2 tablespoons olive oil (30 ml)
- 1 red bell pepper, thinly sliced
- 2 carrots, julienned
- 2 cloves garlic, minced
- 1 tablespoon ginger, minced (15 ml)
- 2 green onions, chopped
- 1/4 cup unsalted peanuts, chopped (60g)
- 2 tablespoons tamari or soy sauce (low sodium) (30 ml)
- 1 tablespoon lime juice (15 ml)
- 1/2 teaspoon red pepper flakes (2.5 ml)
- 1/4 cup fresh cilantro, chopped for garnish (15g)

DIRECTIONS:

1. Preheat the oven to 400°F (200°C). Halve the spaghetti squash lengthwise and remove the seeds. Place cut-side down on a baking sheet and roast until tender, about 30-40 minutes.
2. Once cool enough to handle, use a fork to scrape the squash strands into a bowl, setting them aside.
3. Heat olive oil in a large skillet over medium heat. Add red bell pepper, carrots, garlic, and ginger. Sauté until vegetables are just tender, about 5-7 minutes.
4. Add the spaghetti squash strands to the skillet along with the tamari, lime juice, and red pepper flakes. Toss everything together and cook for an additional 5 minutes to allow flavors to meld.
5. Remove from heat and stir in green onions and peanuts.
6. Serve garnished with fresh cilantro.

NUTRITION INFORMATION: (APPROXIMATE VALUES PER SERVING): Carbohydrates: 28g | Sodium: 280mg | Fats: 9g | Potassium: 350mg | Sugar: 8g | Cholesterol: 0mg

SPICY TOFU AND BOK CHOY STIR-FRY

This Spicy Tofu and Bok Choy Stir-Fry is a quick and flavorful dish packed with protein and fiber, making it an excellent choice for a fatty liver diet.

Prep Time: 10 minutes
Cooking Time: 15 minutes
Complexity: Beginner
Servings: 4
Ingredients: 9

EQUIPMENT NEEDED: Wok or large skillet, spatula, knife, cutting board
TAGS: Whole Foods, vegan, gluten-free, High-protein, High-fiber, Low Sodium, Heart-Healthy, Low Glycemic

INGREDIENT LIST:

- 14 oz firm tofu, pressed and cubed (about 400g)
- 2 tablespoons olive oil (30 ml)
- 2 cloves garlic, minced
- 1 tablespoon fresh ginger, minced (15 ml)
- 4 cups chopped bok choy (about 400g)
- 1 red bell pepper, thinly sliced
- 2 tablespoons gluten-free tamari (30 ml)
- 1 tablespoon chili sauce (15 ml)
- 1 teaspoon sesame oil (5 ml)

DIRECTIONS:

1. Heat olive oil in a wok or large skillet over medium-high heat.
2. Add garlic and ginger, sautéing until fragrant, about 1 minute.
3. Add tofu cubes to the wok and stir-fry until golden, about 5-7 minutes.
4. Incorporate the bok choy and red bell pepper, cooking until the vegetables are tender but still crisp, about 5 minutes.
5. Pour in the tamari and chili sauce, mixing well to coat all ingredients.
6. Drizzle sesame oil over the stir-fry and toss to combine.
7. Serve hot, garnished with sesame seeds or chopped green onions if desired.

NUTRITION INFORMATION: (APPROXIMATE VALUES PER SERVING): Carbohydrates: 10g | Sodium: 320mg | Fats: 14g | Potassium: 300mg | Sugar: 3g | Cholesterol: 0mg

GRILLED HALIBUT WITH CITRUS SALSA

This Grilled Halibut with Citrus Salsa is a fresh and flavorful dish that combines lean protein with vibrant citrus fruits, making it ideal for supporting a healthy liver.

Prep Time: 15 minutes
Cooking Time: 10 minutes
Complexity: Beginner
Servings: 4
Ingredients: 10

EQUIPMENT NEEDED: Grill or grill pan, mixing bowl, knife, cutting board
TAGS: Whole Foods, Heart-Healthy, High-protein, Low Sodium, Vitamin C rich

INGREDIENT LIST:

- 4 halibut fillets (about 6 oz or 170g each)
- 2 tablespoons olive oil (30 ml)
- Salt and pepper to taste
- 1 orange, peeled and diced
- 1 grapefruit, peeled and diced
- 1 lime, juice and zest
- 1 small red onion, finely chopped 1/4 cup chopped fresh cilantro (15g)
- 1 jalapeño, seeded and finely chopped (optional)
- 1 tablespoon honey (15 ml)

DIRECTIONS:

1. Preheat the grill or grill pan over medium-high heat.
2. Brush the halibut fillets with olive oil and season with salt and pepper.
3. Grill the halibut for about 4-5 minutes on each side, or until the fish flakes easily with a fork.
4. While the fish is grilling, combine the orange, grapefruit, lime juice and zest, red onion, cilantro, jalapeño (if using), and honey in a bowl to make the citrus salsa.
5. Mix the salsa gently to combine the flavors.
6. Serve the grilled halibut topped with a generous amount of citrus salsa.

NUTRITION INFORMATION: (APPROXIMATE VALUES PER SERVING): Carbohydrates: 15g | Sodium: 70mg | Fats: 12g | Potassium: 600mg | Sugar: 10g | Cholesterol: 45mg

MISO-GLAZED COD WITH BOK CHOY

This Miso-Glazed Cod with Bok Choy features a succulent piece of cod with a flavorful miso glaze paired with tender bok choy. This dish is rich in protein and essential vitamins, making it perfect for a healthy liver diet.

Prep Time: 10 minutes
Cooking Time: 15 minutes
Complexity: Intermediate
Servings: 4
Ingredients: 8

EQUIPMENT NEEDED: Baking sheet, small bowl, brush, oven
TAGS: Whole Foods, Heart-Healthy, High-protein, Low Sodium, Low Glycemic, Vitamin C rich

INGREDIENT LIST:

- 4 cod fillets (6 oz each or 170g)
- 2 tablespoons white miso paste (30 ml)
- 1 tablespoon honey (15 ml)
- 1 tablespoon rice vinegar (15 ml)
- 1 teaspoon sesame oil (5 ml)
- 4 baby bok choy, halved
- 1 tablespoon olive oil (15 ml)
- Fresh ground black pepper, to taste

DIRECTIONS:

1. Preheat the oven to 400°F (200°C).
2. In a small bowl, mix the miso paste, honey, rice vinegar, and sesame oil until smooth.
3. Place the cod fillets on a greased baking sheet.
4. Brush the miso mixture over each fillet evenly.
5. Toss the bok choy halves in olive oil and arrange them around the cod on the baking sheet. Sprinkle with black pepper.
6. Bake in the preheated oven for about 12-15 minutes or until the cod is opaque and flakes easily with a fork.
7. Serve the miso-glazed cod with the roasted bok choy on the side.

NUTRITION INFORMATION: (APPROXIMATE VALUES PER SERVING): Carbohydrates: 12g | Sodium: 290mg | Fats: 8g | Potassium: 650mg | Sugar: 5g | Cholesterol: 60mg

ROASTED BRUSSELS SPROUTS AND POMEGRANATE SALAD

This vibrant salad combines roasted Brussels sprouts with juicy pomegranate seeds, delivering a dish rich in fiber, vitamins, and antioxidants, perfect for a healthy liver diet.

Prep Time: 10 minutes
Cooking Time: 20 minutes
Complexity: Beginner
Servings: 4
Ingredients: 6

EQUIPMENT NEEDED: Oven, baking sheet, mixing bowl, knife, cutting board
TAGS: Whole Foods, vegan, Heart-Healthy, High-fiber, Low Sodium, Vitamin C rich, Vitamin E rich

INGREDIENT LIST:

- 1 lb Brussels sprouts, halved (about 450g)
- 2 tablespoons olive oil (30 ml)
- Salt and pepper to taste
- 1/2 cup pomegranate seeds (about 88g)
- 1/4 cup chopped walnuts (30g)
- 1 tablespoon balsamic vinegar (15 ml)

DIRECTIONS:

1. Preheat the oven to 400°F (200°C).
2. Toss the halved Brussels sprouts with olive oil, salt, and pepper. Spread them on a baking sheet.
3. Roast in the preheated oven for 20 minutes or until crisp on the outside and tender on the inside.
4. Remove the Brussels sprouts from the oven and let them cool slightly.
5. In a large bowl, combine the roasted Brussels sprouts with pomegranate seeds and chopped walnuts.
6. Drizzle with balsamic vinegar and toss to coat evenly.
7. Serve the salad warm or at room temperature.

NUTRITION INFORMATION: (APPROXIMATE VALUES PER SERVING): Carbohydrates: 18g | Sodium: 30mg | Fats: 12g | Potassium: 450mg | Sugar: 7g | Cholesterol: 0mg

SEARED SCALLOPS WITH QUINOA AND APPLE SALAD

This dish combines seared scallops with refreshing quinoa and apple salad, providing a nutritious meal rich in protein and fibe while being low in sodium and fats, suitable for those managing fatty liver disease.

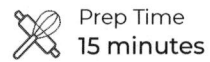

Prep Time: 15 minutes | **Cooking Time:** 10 minutes | **Complexity:** Intermediate | **Servings:** 4 | **Ingredients:** 9

EQUIPMENT NEEDED: Skillet, mixing bowl, spoon, knife, cutting board
TAGS: Whole Foods, Heart-Healthy, High-protein, High-fiber, Low Sodium, gluten-free

INGREDIENT LIST:

- 12 large scallops (about 1 lb or 450g)
- 1 tablespoon olive oil (15 ml)
- 1 cup quinoa, cooked (about 185g)
- 1 large apple, diced
- 1/4 cup dried cranberries (about 30g)
- 1/4 cup chopped walnuts (30g)
- 2 tablespoons lemon juice (30 ml)
- 1/2 teaspoon black pepper (2.5 ml)
- Salt to taste

DIRECTIONS:

1. Heat olive oil in a skillet over medium-high heat.
2. Pat scallops dry with a paper towel and season lightly with sal and pepper.
3. Sear the scallops for about 2 minutes on each side until golder brown and cooked through.
4. In a mixing bowl, combine the cooked quinoa, diced apple dried cranberries, and chopped walnuts.
5. Dress the quinoa salad with lemon juice, season with blacl pepper, and mix well.
6. Serve the seared scallops over the quinoa and apple salad.

NUTRITION INFORMATION: (APPROXIMATE VALUES PER SERVING): Carbohydrates: 35g | Sodium: 180mg | Fats: 10g | Potassium: 520mg | Sugar: 12g | Cholesterol: 37mg

HERB ROASTED CHICKEN WITH ROOT VEGETABLES

This wholesome dish features herb-roasted chicken accompanied by a medley of root vegetables, offering a nutritious meal that's high in protein and fiber, and low in sodium, perfectly aligned with a fatty liver diet.

Prep Time: 20 minutes | **Cooking Time:** 50 minutes | **Complexity:** Intermediate | **Servings:** 4 | **Ingredients:** 9

EQUIPMENT NEEDED: Roasting pan, knife, cutting board, mixing bowl, measuring spoons
TAGS: Whole Foods, Heart-Healthy, High-protein, High-fiber, Low Sodium, gluten-free, Vitamin A rich, Vitamin C rich

INGREDIENT LIST:

- 4 skinless chicken breasts (about 6 oz or 170g each)
- 2 tablespoons olive oil (30 ml)
- 1 teaspoon dried rosemary (5 ml)
- 1 teaspoon dried thyme (5 ml)
- 2 carrots, peeled and chopped
- 2 parsnips, peeled and chopped
- 1 sweet potato, peeled and cubed
- 1 onion, peeled and quartered
- Salt and pepper to taste

DIRECTIONS:

1. Preheat the oven to 375°F (190°C).
2. In a large bowl, mix the olive oil, rosemary, thyme, salt, and pep per.
3. Toss the chicken breasts and all the chopped vegetables in the herb-oil mixture until well-coated.
4. Arrange the chicken and vegetables in a single layer on a roast ing pan.
5. Roast in the preheated oven for about 45-50 minutes, or unti the chicken is cooked through and the vegetables are tende and golden.
6. Remove from the oven and let rest for a few minutes before serving to allow the juices to redistribute.

NUTRITION INFORMATION: (APPROXIMATE VALUES PER SERVING): Carbohydrates: 22g | Sodium: 150mg | Fats: 16g | Potassium: 600mg | Sugar: 6g | Cholesterol: 75mg

PUMPKIN CURRY WITH BROWN RICE

This Pumpkin Curry with Brown Rice is a hearty, comforting meal that perfectly fits into a fatty liver diet. It combines the richness of pumpkin with the wholesomeness of brown rice, making it a nutrient-packed dinner option.

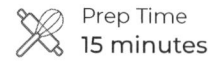

Prep Time: 15 minutes
Cooking Time: 30 minutes
Complexity: Beginner
Servings: 4
Ingredients: 10

EQUIPMENT NEEDED: Large pot, skillet, wooden spoon, knife, cutting board

TAGS: Whole Foods, vegan, Heart-Healthy, High-fiber, Low Sodium, Low Glycemic, Vitamin A rich, Vitamin C rich

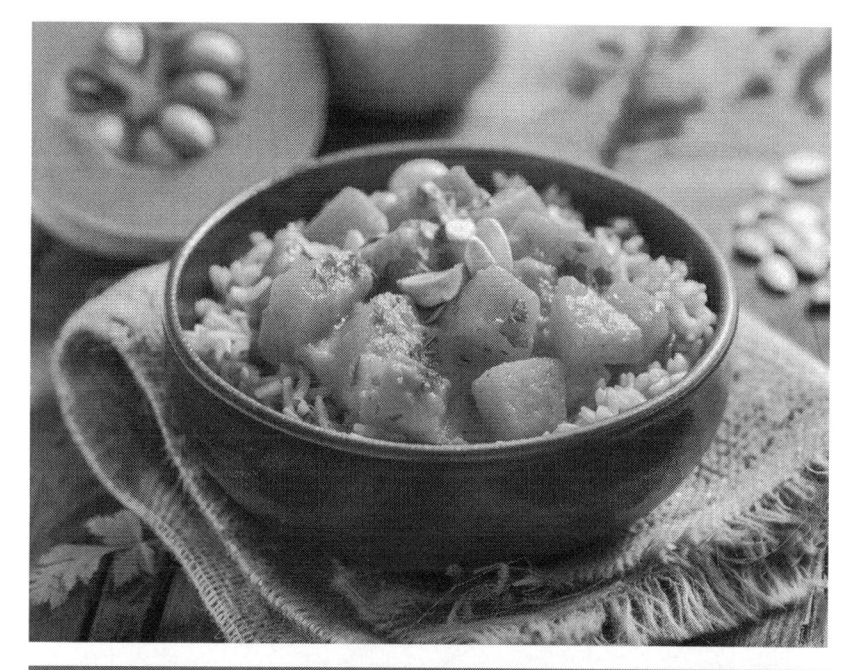

INGREDIENT LIST:

- 1 cup brown rice (190g), rinsed
- 2 cups water (475 ml) for cooking rice
- 1 tablespoon olive oil (15 ml)
- 1 onion, chopped
- 2 cloves garlic, minced
- 2 cups pumpkin, peeled and cubed (about 300g)
- 1 can (14 oz or 400 ml) coconut milk
- 1 tablespoon curry powder (15 ml)
- 1 teaspoon turmeric (5 ml)
- Salt to taste
- Fresh cilantro, chopped for garnish

DIRECTIONS:

1. In a medium pot, bring 2 cups of water to a boil. Add the brown rice, reduce heat to low, cover, and simmer for about 25-30 minutes, or until the water is absorbed and the rice is tender.
2. Meanwhile, heat the olive oil in a large skillet over medium heat. Add the onion and garlic, and sauté until the onion becomes translucent.
3. Add the pumpkin cubes to the skillet and cook for about 5 minutes, stirring occasionally.
4. Stir in the coconut milk, curry powder, and turmeric. Reduce the heat and let the curry simmer for about 15 minutes, or until the pumpkin is tender and the curry has thickened.
5. Season with salt to taste.
6. Serve the pumpkin curry over the cooked brown rice, garnished with chopped cilantro.

NUTRITION INFORMATION: (APPROXIMATE VALUES PER SERVING): Carbohydrates: 50g | Sodium: 50mg | Fats: 14g | Potassium: 600mg | Sugar: 5g | Cholesterol: 0mg

VEGAN MUSHROOM AND LENTIL BOLOGNESE

This Vegan Mushroom and Lentil Bolognese is a hearty, nutritious dish that mimics the texture and flavor of traditional meat sauces while being completely plant-based. It's rich in protein and fiber, making it ideal for those on a fatty liver diet.

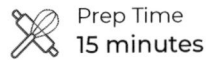

Prep Time: 15 minutes
Cooking Time: 30 minutes
Complexity: Intermediate
Servings: 4
Ingredients: 10

EQUIPMENT NEEDED: Large skillet, saucepan, wooden spoon, knife, cutting board
TAGS: Whole Foods, vegan, Heart-Healthy, High-fiber, Low Sodium, gluten-free, High-protein

INGREDIENT LIST:

- 1 cup brown lentils (190g), rinsed and drained
- 2 tablespoons olive oil (30 ml)
- 1 large onion, finely chopped
- 2 cloves garlic, minced
- 2 cups mushrooms, chopped (about 150g), 1 carrot, finely diced
- 1 celery stalk, finely diced
- 1 can (28 oz or 800g) crushed tomatoes, 2 teaspoons dried Italian herbs (10 ml)
- Salt and pepper to taste
- Fresh basil, chopped (for garnish)

DIRECTIONS:

1. Cook lentils in a saucepan with enough water to cover them by a few inches. Bring to a boil, then simmer for 20-25 minutes or until tender. Drain any excess water.
2. While the lentils are cooking, heat the olive oil in a large skillet over medium heat.
3. Add the onion and garlic, sautéing until the onion becomes translucent.
4. Add the mushrooms, carrot, and celery to the skillet. Cook until the vegetables are softened, about 8-10 minutes.
5. Stir in the cooked lentils, crushed tomatoes, and dried Italian herbs. Season with salt and pepper.
6. Reduce heat to low and let the sauce simmer for about 10 minutes, allowing the flavors to meld.
7. Serve hot cooked whole grain pasta or a bed of steamed vegetables, garnished with fresh basil.

NUTRITION INFORMATION: (APPROXIMATE VALUES PER SERVING): Carbohydrates: 45g | Sodium: 300mg | Fats: 9g | Potassium: 800mg | Sugar: 8g | Cholesterol: 0mg

LEMON AND HERB POACHED HADDOCK

This Lemon and Herb Poached Haddock is a light and flavorful dish, perfect for those on a fatty liver diet. It pairs the delicate taste of haddock with aromatic herbs and lemon, creating a meal that's both nutritious and satisfying.

Prep Time: 10 minutes
Cooking Time: 15 minutes
Complexity: Beginner
Servings: 4
Ingredients: 7

EQUIPMENT NEEDED: Skillet, lid, measuring spoons, knife, cutting board
TAGS: Whole Foods, Heart-Healthy, High-protein, Low Sodium, Low Fat, Vitamin C rich, gluten-free, dairy-free

INGREDIENT LIST:

- 4 haddock fillets (about 6 oz or 170g each)
- 2 tablespoons olive oil (30 ml)
- Juice and zest of 1 lemon
- 1 cup low-sodium vegetable broth (240 ml)
- 1 tablespoon fresh dill, chopped (15 ml)
- 1 tablespoon fresh parsley, chopped (15 ml)
- Salt and pepper to taste

DIRECTIONS:

1. Heat olive oil in a skillet over medium heat.
2. Place the haddock fillets in the skillet.
3. Add the lemon juice, lemon zest, and vegetable broth. The liquid should just about cover the fillets.
4. Sprinkle the chopped dill and parsley over the fillets.
5. Season with salt and pepper to taste.
6. Bring the liquid to a simmer, then reduce the heat to low. Cover and let poach gently for about 10-12 minutes, or until the haddock is opaque and flakes easily with a fork.
7. Carefully remove the haddock from the skillet and serve with a drizzle of the cooking liquid and additional herbs if desired.

NUTRITION INFORMATION: (APPROXIMATE VALUES PER SERVING): Carbohydrates: 2g | Sodium: 70mg | Fats: 9g | Potassium: 500mg | Sugar: 0g | Cholesterol: 60mg

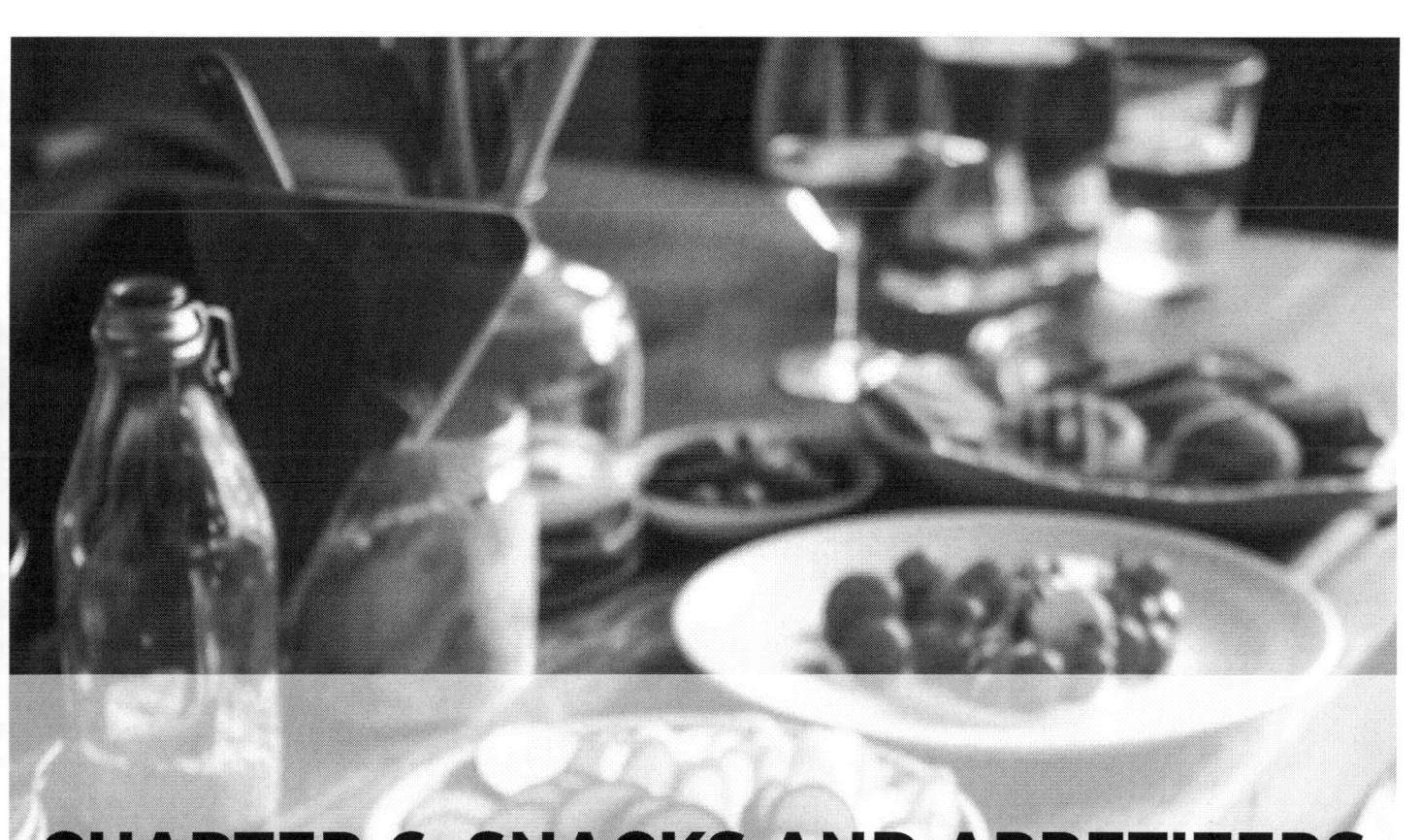

CHAPTER 6: SNACKS AND APPETIZERS

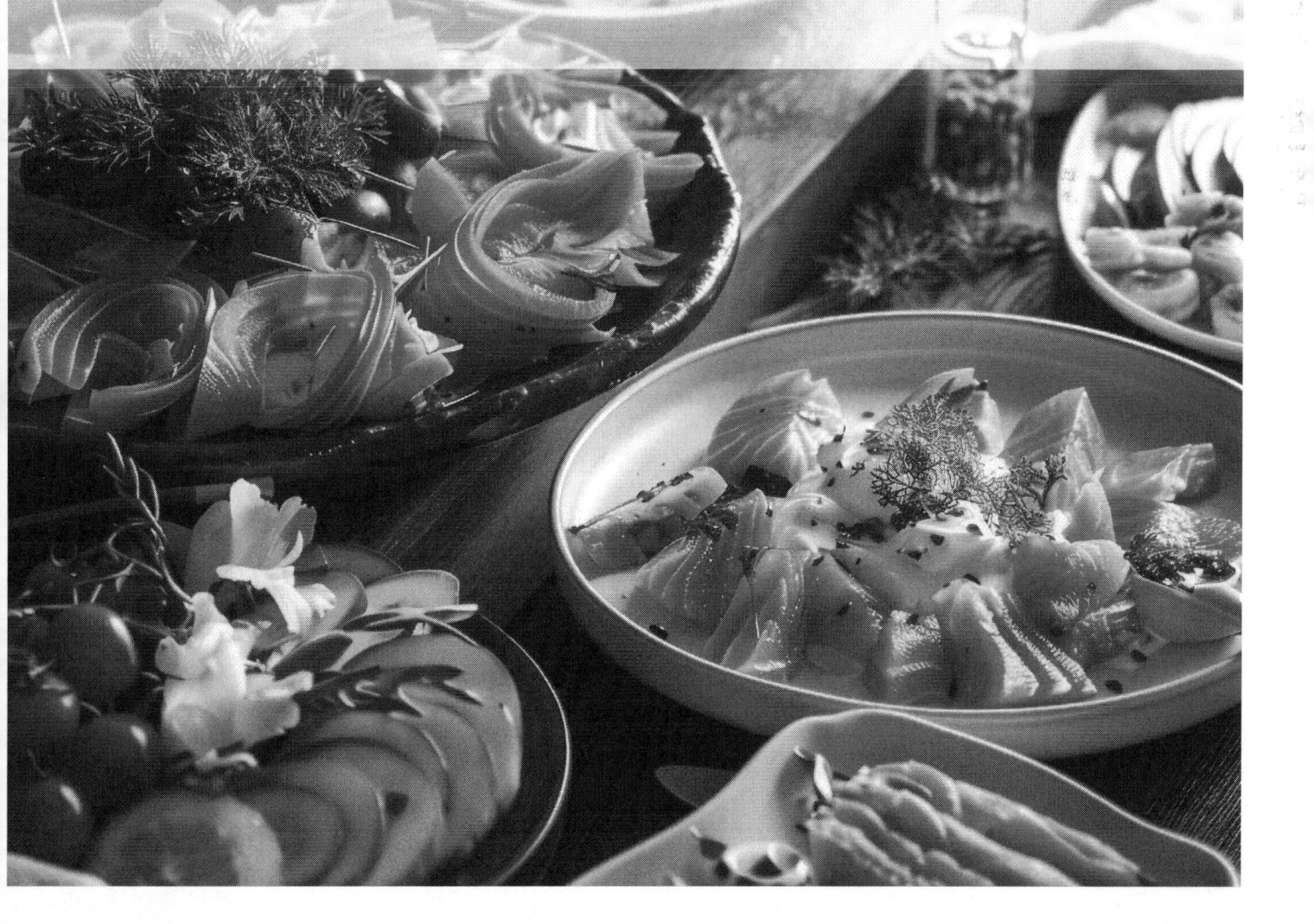

AIR-FRIED SPICED CARROT CHIPS

These Air-Fried Spiced Carrot Chips are a crunchy, delicious alternative to traditional snacks. Perfectly aligned with a fatty liver diet, they offer a great way to enjoy a low-calorie, high-fiber snack that's easy on the liver and delightful on the palate.

- **Prep Time:** 10 minutes
- **Cooking Time:** 15 minutes
- **Complexity:** Beginner
- **Servings:** 4
- **Ingredients:** 5

EQUIPMENT NEEDED: Air fryer, knife, cutting board, mixing bowl, measuring spoons

TAGS: Whole Foods, vegan, gluten-free, dairy-free, Low Glycemic, Heart-Healthy, High-fiber, Low Sodium, low-fat, low-calorie, Vitamin A rich

INGREDIENT LIST:

- 4 large carrots, peeled and thinly sliced (about 600g)
- 1 tablespoon olive oil (15 ml)
- 1/2 teaspoon paprika (2.5 ml)
- 1/4 teaspoon ground cumin (1.25 ml)
- Salt to taste

DIRECTIONS:

1. In a mixing bowl, toss the thinly sliced carrots with olive oil, paprika, cumin, and a pinch of salt to ensure they are evenly coated.
2. Preheat the air fryer to 360°F (182°C).
3. Arrange the carrot slices in a single layer in the air fryer basket, ensuring they don't overlap to promote even cooking.
4. Air fry for about 15 minutes, or until crisp and golden, shaking the basket halfway through cooking.
5. Remove the carrot chips from the air fryer and let them cool slightly; they will continue to crisp up as they cool.
6. Serve immediately for the best texture, or store in an airtight container once fully cooled.

NUTRITION INFORMATION: (APPROXIMATE VALUES PER SERVING): Carbohydrates: 9g | Sodium: 50mg | Fats: 3.5g | Potassium: 290mg | Sugar: 5g | Cholesterol: 0mg

SMOKED SALMON AND CREAM CHEESE CUCUMBER ROLLS

These Smoked Salmon and Cream Cheese Cucumber Rolls are a light and refreshing appetizer, perfect for a fatty liver diet. They combine the lean protein of smoked salmon with the freshness of cucumber, offering a delicious, heart-healthy snack.

- **Prep Time:** 15 minutes
- **Cooking Time:** 0 minutes
- **Complexity:** Beginner
- **Servings:** 4
- **Ingredients:** 5

EQUIPMENT NEEDED: Vegetable peeler, knife, mixing bowl, spoon

TAGS: Whole Foods, Heart-Healthy, High-protein, Low Sodium, Low Fat, gluten-free, dairy-free, low-calorie, Vitamin D rich, Vitamin E rich

INGREDIENT LIST:

- 2 large cucumbers
- 8 oz smoked salmon, thinly sliced (about 225g)
- 4 oz low-fat cream cheese, softened (about 113g)
- 1 tablespoon capers, rinsed and chopped (15 ml)
- Fresh dill for garnish

DIRECTIONS:

1. Using a vegetable peeler, slice the cucumbers lengthwise into thin strips.
2. Lay out the cucumber strips on a clean surface.
3. Spread a thin layer of cream cheese over each cucumber strip.
4. Place a slice of smoked salmon on top of the cream cheese on each cucumber strip.
5. Sprinkle chopped capers evenly over the salmon.
6. Carefully roll up each cucumber strip tightly.
7. Garnish with fresh dill.
8. Serve immediately, or chill in the refrigerator until ready to serve.

NUTRITION INFORMATION: (APPROXIMATE VALUES PER SERVING): Carbohydrates: 5g | Sodium: 200mg | Fats: 7g | Potassium: 300mg | Sugar: 2g | Cholesterol: 20mg

CUCUMBER BOATS WITH SPICY SHRIMP SALAD

This appetizing dish combines the freshness of cucumber with a spicy shrimp salad, making a perfect snack or appetizer that aligns with a fatty liver diet by being high in protein, low in sodium, and rich in essential nutrients.

- **Prep Time:** 15 minutes
- **Cooking Time:** 5 minutes
- **Complexity:** Beginner
- **Servings:** 4
- **Ingredients:** 8

EQUIPMENT NEEDED: Knife, cutting board, mixing bowl, spoon

TAGS: Whole Foods, Heart-Healthy, High-protein, Low Sodium, Low Fat, gluten-free, dairy-free, low-calorie, Vitamin C rich

INGREDIENT LIST:

- 2 large cucumbers
- 8 oz (225g) shrimp, peeled and deveined
- 1 tablespoon olive oil (15 ml)
- 1 teaspoon chili flakes (5 ml) or to taste
- Juice of 1 lime
- 1 tablespoon chopped fresh cilantro (15 ml)
- 1/4 red onion, finely chopped
- Salt and pepper to taste

DIRECTIONS:

1. In a skillet over medium heat, add the olive oil and shrimp. Season with salt, pepper, and chili flakes.
2. Cook the shrimp for 2-3 minutes on each side until pink and fully cooked. Remove from heat and let cool slightly.
3. Once cooled, chop the shrimp into small pieces and place in a mixing bowl.
4. Add the lime juice, chopped cilantro, and red onion to the shrimp. Stir to combine all ingredients thoroughly.
5. Cut the cucumbers in half lengthwise and scoop out the seeds with a spoon to create a hollow boat.
6. Fill each cucumber boat with the spicy shrimp salad mixture.
7. Serve immediately or chill in the refrigerator before serving to enhance the flavors.

NUTRITION INFORMATION: (APPROXIMATE VALUES PER SERVING): Carbohydrates: 4g | Sodium: 85mg | Fats: 7g | Potassium: 200mg | Sugar: 2g | Cholesterol: 85mg

ROASTED BRUSSELS SPROUTS WITH LEMON DIP

This dish pairs perfectly roasted Brussels sprouts with a tangy lemon dip, creating a delightful appetizer that adheres to a fatty liver diet by being low in sodium, rich in fiber, and packed with nutrients.

- **Prep Time:** 10 minutes
- **Cooking Time:** 25 minutes
- **Complexity:** Beginner
- **Servings:** 4
- **Ingredients:** 7

EQUIPMENT NEEDED: Oven, baking sheet, mixing bowl, whisk, knife, cutting board

TAGS: Whole Foods, Heart-Healthy, High-fiber, Low Sodium, gluten-free, dairy-free, Low Fat, low-calorie, Vitamin C rich, Vegan

INGREDIENT LIST:

- 1 lb (450g) Brussels sprouts, trimmed and halved
- 2 tablespoons olive oil (30 ml)
- Salt and pepper to taste
- 1 cup plain low-fat yogurt (240 ml) [for a vegan version, use a plant-based yogurt]
- Zest and juice of 1 lemon
- 1 tablespoon Dijon mustard (15 ml)
- 1 garlic clove, minced

DIRECTIONS:

1. Preheat your oven to 400°F (200°C). In a large bowl, toss the Brussels sprouts with olive oil, salt, and pepper.
2. Spread the Brussels sprouts on a baking sheet in a single layer.
3. Roast in the preheated oven for about 25 minutes, or until crispy on the outside and tender on the inside, stirring halfway through for even cooking.
4. While the Brussels sprouts are roasting, prepare the lemon dip. In a small bowl, combine the yogurt, lemon zest, lemon juice, Dijon mustard, and minced garlic. Whisk until smooth and creamy. Season the dip with salt and pepper to taste.
5. Serve the roasted Brussels sprouts warm with the lemon dip on the side.

NUTRITION INFORMATION: (APPROXIMATE VALUES PER SERVING): Carbohydrates: 15g | Sodium: 125mg | Fats: 8g | Potassium: 440mg | Sugar: 4g | Cholesterol: 2mg

RICOTTA AND BERRY STUFFED CELERY

This delightful snack pairs the crispness of celery with the creamy texture of ricotta cheese and the sweet burst of berries, creating a nutritious and tasty option perfect for adhering to a fatty liver diet.

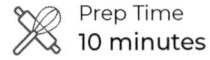

Prep Time: 10 minutes
Cooking Time: 0 minutes
Complexity: Beginner
Servings: 4
Ingredients: 4

EQUIPMENT NEEDED: Knife, mixing bowl, spoon

TAGS: Whole Foods, vegetarian, gluten-free, Low Glycemic, Heart-Healthy, High-fiber, Low Sodium, low-fat, low-calorie, Vitamin C rich

INGREDIENT LIST:

- 8 large celery stalks
- 1 cup low-fat ricotta cheese (240 ml)
- 1/2 cup mixed berries (blueberries, raspberries, chopped strawberries) (about 75g)
- Fresh mint leaves, chopped (for garnish)

DIRECTIONS:

1. Wash the celery stalks and pat them dry. Cut each stalk into 3-4 inch long pieces.
2. In a mixing bowl, combine the ricotta cheese with the mixed berries, gently folding to incorporate without crushing the berries.
3. Using a spoon, fill each celery piece with the ricotta and berry mixture.
4. Garnish each stuffed celery with chopped mint leaves for added flavor and a touch of color.
5. Serve immediately or chill in the refrigerator before serving for a refreshing snack.

NUTRITION INFORMATION: (APPROXIMATE VALUES PER SERVING): Carbohydrates: 8g | Sodium: 80mg | Fats: 3g | Potassium: 200mg | Sugar: 4g | Cholesterol: 10mg

ZUCCHINI AND HERB FRITTERS

These Zucchini and Herb Fritters are a savory, nutritious snack that combines the freshness of zucchini with aromatic herbs, ideal for a fatty liver diet. They are baked instead of fried, providing a healthier option that's low in fat and high in fiber.

Prep Time: 10 minutes
Cooking Time: 20 minutes
Complexity: Beginner
Servings: 4
Ingredients: 7

EQUIPMENT NEEDED: Oven, mixing bowl, grater, baking sheet, parchment paper, spoon

TAGS: Whole Foods, vegetarian, gluten-free, High-fiber, Low Sodium, low-fat, low-calorie, Heart-Healthy

INGREDIENT LIST:

- 2 medium zucchinis, grated
- 1/2 cup almond flour (or any gluten-free flour) (60 ml)
- 2 eggs, beaten
- 1/4 cup chopped fresh herbs (parsley, dill, and chives) (60 ml)
- 1 garlic clove, minced
- Salt and pepper to taste
- Olive oil spray (for baking)

DIRECTIONS:

1. Preheat the oven to 400°F (200°C). Line a baking sheet with parchment paper and lightly spray with olive oil.
2. Place the grated zucchini in a colander, sprinkle with a little salt, and let it sit for 10 minutes. Squeeze out as much liquid as possible.
3. In a mixing bowl, combine the drained zucchini, almond flour, beaten eggs, chopped herbs, minced garlic, salt, and pepper. Mix well to form a cohesive batter.
4. Scoop tablespoons of the batter onto the prepared baking sheet, flattening them slightly to form fritters.
5. Spray the tops of the fritters lightly with olive oil.
6. Bake in the preheated oven for 10 minutes, then flip the fritters and bake for an additional 10 minutes or until golden and crispy.
7. Serve warm with a side of low-fat yogurt or a light sour cream dip if desired.

NUTRITION INFORMATION: (APPROXIMATE VALUES PER SERVING): Carbohydrates: 8g | Sodium: 80mg | Fats: 7g | Potassium: 300mg | Sugar: 4g | Cholesterol: 95mg

BAKED COD FISH STICKS WITH YOGURT DILL SAUCE

These Baked Cod Fish Sticks with Yogurt Dill Sauce provide a delightful twist on the traditional fish stick, offering a healthy, protein-rich option that is baked instead of fried to reduce fat content, aligning with a fatty liver diet.

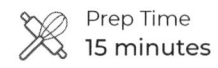

Prep Time: 15 minutes
Cooking Time: 20 minutes
Complexity: Beginner
Servings: 4
Ingredients: 10

EQUIPMENT NEEDED: Oven, baking sheet, mixing bowls, whisk, knife, cutting board

TAGS: Heart-Healthy, High-protein, Low Sodium, low-fat, low-calorie, gluten-free, High-fiber, Vitamin D-rich

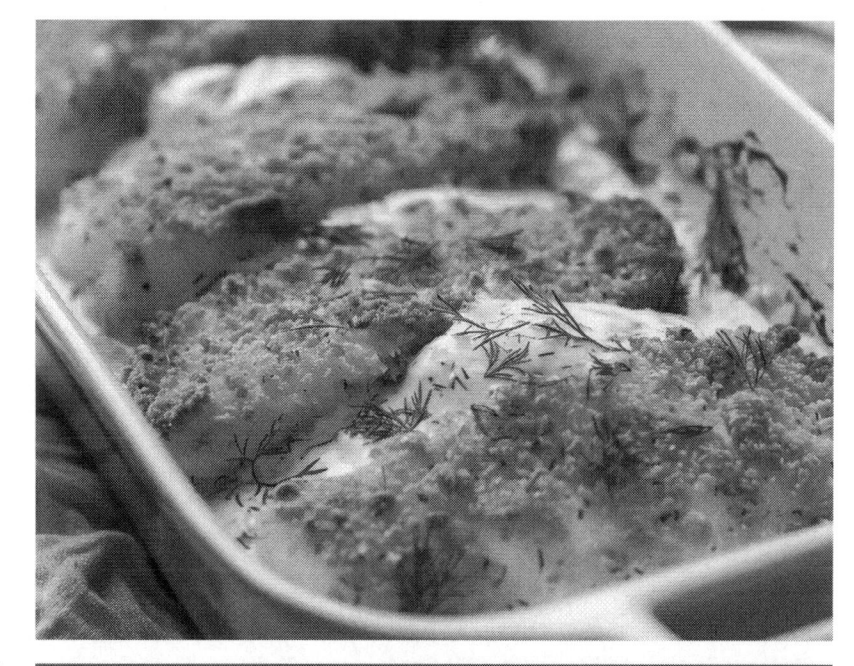

INGREDIENT LIST:

- 1 lb (450g) cod fillets, cut into strips
- 1 cup gluten-free breadcrumbs
- 1/2 cup grated Parmesan cheese (optional for dairy-free, omit if necessary)
- 1 teaspoon paprika
- 1/2 teaspoon garlic powder
- Salt and pepper to taste
- 2 eggs, beaten
- Olive oil spray
- 1 cup plain Greek yogurt (use dairy-free yogurt for a dairy-free option)
- 2 tablespoons fresh dill, chopped
- Juice of 1 lemon

DIRECTIONS:

1. Preheat your oven to 400°F (200°C). Line a baking sheet with parchment paper and lightly spray with olive oil.
2. In a shallow bowl, combine the gluten-free breadcrumbs, grated Parmesan (if using), paprika, garlic powder, salt, and pepper.
3. Place the beaten eggs in another shallow bowl.
4. Dip each cod strip first in the beaten eggs, then coat evenly with the breadcrumb mixture.
5. Arrange the breaded cod strips on the prepared baking sheet. Spray lightly with olive oil.
6. Bake in the preheated oven for 20 minutes, turning halfway through, until the fish is cooked through and the coating is golden and crispy.
7. While the fish bake, prepare the yogurt dill sauce: In a small bowl, whisk together the Greek yogurt, chopped dill, and lemon juice. Season with salt and pepper to taste.
8. Serve the baked fish sticks hot with the yogurt dill sauce on the side.

NUTRITION INFORMATION: (APPROXIMATE VALUES PER SERVING): Carbohydrates: 18g | Sodium: 240mg | Fats: 9g | Potassium: 460mg | Sugar: 3g | Cholesterol: 120mg

PUMPKIN HUMMUS WITH WHOLE GRAIN PITA CHIPS

This Pumpkin Hummus with Whole Grain Pita Chips is a delicious and nutritious snack that blends the sweet, earthy flavors of pumpkin with the creamy texture of hummus, complemented by crispy whole-grain pita chips.

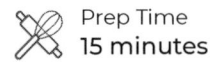

Prep Time: 15 minutes
Cooking Time: 10 minutes
Complexity: Beginner
Servings: 4
Ingredients: 9

EQUIPMENT NEEDED: Oven, food processor, baking sheet, mixing bowl, knife
TAGS: Whole Foods, vegetarian, gluten-free, High-fiber, Low Sodium, low-fat, low-calorie, Heart-Healthy, Vitamin A rich, Vitamin C rich

INGREDIENT LIST:

- 1 can (15 oz) chickpeas, drained and rinsed
- 1 cup canned pumpkin puree (not pie filling)
- 2 tablespoons tahini
- 2 cloves garlic, minced
- Juice of 1 lemon
- 1/2 teaspoon ground cumin
- Salt and pepper to taste
- Whole grain pita bread, cut into triangles
- Olive oil spray

DIRECTIONS:

1. Preheat your oven to 375°F (190°C). Arrange the pita triangles on a baking sheet and lightly spray with olive oil. Season with a pinch of salt if desired.
2. Bake the pita chips in the preheated oven for about 10 minutes or until crispy and golden. Set aside to cool.
3. In a food processor, combine the chickpeas, pumpkin puree, tahini, minced garlic, lemon juice, ground cumin, salt, and pepper. Blend until smooth.
4. If the hummus is too thick, add a little water or additional lemon juice to reach the desired consistency.
5. Taste and adjust seasoning as needed.
6. Serve the pumpkin hummus in a bowl, accompanied by the baked whole-grain pita chips.

NUTRITION INFORMATION: (APPROXIMATE VALUES PER SERVING): Carbohydrates: 35g | Sodium: 200mg | Fats: 5g | Potassium: 250mg | Sugar: 4g | Cholesterol: 0mg

KALE AND APPLE CHIPS

This snack offers a delightful crunch and nutritional richness, perfect for adhering to a fatty liver diet. Kale and Apple Chips are not only delicious but also packed with fiber, vitamins, and minerals, making them an excellent low-calorie, heart-healthy option.

Prep Time: 10 minutes
Cooking Time: 20 minutes
Complexity: Beginner
Servings: 4
Ingredients: 4

EQUIPMENT NEEDED: Oven, baking sheet, knife, mixing bowl
TAGS: Whole Foods, vegan, gluten-free, dairy-free, Low Glycemic, Heart-Healthy, High-fiber, Low Sodium, low-fat, low-calorie, Vitamin A rich, Vitamin C rich

INGREDIENT LIST:

- 1 large bunch of kale, leaves torn from stems and chopped
- 2 large apples, thinly sliced
- 1 tablespoon olive oil
- Salt to taste (optional)

DIRECTIONS:

1. Preheat your oven to 300°F (150°C). Line two baking sheets with parchment paper. In a mixing bowl, toss the kale leaves with half of the olive oil. Spread the leaves in a single layer on one of the baking sheets. Sprinkle lightly with salt if desired.
2. In the same bowl, toss the apple slices with the remaining olive oil. Spread the apple slices in a single layer on the second baking sheet.
3. Bake in the preheated oven for 20 minutes or until the kale is crispy and the apple slices are dried out but still pliable. Check frequently to avoid burning, as oven temperatures may vary.
4. Allow the chips to cool on the baking sheets to maintain crispness.

NUTRITION INFORMATION: (APPROXIMATE VALUES PER SERVING): Carbohydrates: 15g | Sodium: 50mg | Fats: 3g | Potassium: 300mg | Sugar: 10g | Cholesterol: 0mg

TAHINI AND COCOA ENERGY BITES

These energy bites are a delicious and nutritious snack that supports liver health with healthy fats, high protein, and fiber content. They're perfect for a quick energy boost without the added sugars, making them ideal for managing a fatty liver.

Prep Time: 15 minutes
Cooking Time: 0 minutes
Complexity: Beginner
Servings: 12
Ingredients: 6

EQUIPMENT NEEDED: Mixing bowl, spoon, measuring cups, refrigerator

TAGS: Whole Foods, vegan, gluten-free, dairy-free, High-protein, High-fiber, Low Sodium, low-fat, low-calorie, Heart-Healthy, Low Glycemic, Sugar-Free

INGREDIENT LIST:

- 1 cup (240 ml) tahini
- 1/4 cup (60 ml) cocoa powder, unsweetened
- 1/2 cup (120 ml) ground flaxseed
- 1/4 cup (60 ml) unsweetened shredded coconut
- 2 tablespoons (30 ml) honey (substitute with agave syrup for a vegan option)
- A pinch of salt (optional)

DIRECTIONS:

1. In a mixing bowl, combine tahini and cocoa powder until well blended.
2. Stir in ground flaxseed, shredded coconut, honey (or agave syrup), and a pinch of salt if using. Mix until the mixture is uniform and sticks together.
3. Using your hands, roll the mixture into small balls about the size of a walnut.
4. Place the rolled energy bites on a plate or tray and refrigerate for at least 30 minutes to set.
5. Keep the energy bites refrigerated in an airtight container for up to one week.

NUTRITION INFORMATION: (APPROXIMATE VALUES PER SERVING): Carbohydrates: 8g | Sodium: 15mg | Fats: 14g | Potassium: 200mg | Sugar: 3g | Cholesterol: 0mg

STUFFED CHERRY TOMATOES WITH TUNA SALAD

Enjoy a refreshing and nutritious snack with these stuffed cherry tomatoes filled with a hearty tuna salad. This recipe combines lean protein, healthy fats, and low-sodium ingredients, making it a perfect choice for anyone following a fatty liver diet.

Prep Time: 15 minutes
Cooking Time: 0 minutes
Complexity: Beginner
Servings: 4
Ingredients: 7

EQUIPMENT NEEDED: Bowl, knife, spoon

TAGS: High-protein, Low Sodium, low-fat, High-fiber, Heart-Healthy, Low Glycemic, Sugar-Free, gluten-free, Vitamin C rich

INGREDIENT LIST:

- 16 large cherry tomatoes (approx. 1 pint)
- 1 can (6 ounces or 170 g) no-salt-added tuna, drained
- 1/4 cup (60 ml) low-fat Greek yogurt
- 1 tablespoon (15 ml) Dijon mustard
- 1 tablespoon (15 ml) chopped fresh parsley
- 1/4 teaspoon (1.25 ml) black pepper
- 2 tablespoons (30 ml) finely chopped celery

DIRECTIONS:

1. Slice the tops off the cherry tomatoes and carefully scoop out the seeds with a small spoon or melon baller to create a hollow center. Set aside the hollowed tomatoes.
2. In a bowl, combine the drained tuna, Greek yogurt, Dijon mustard, chopped parsley, black pepper, and chopped celery. Mix thoroughly to create a smooth and even tuna salad.
3. Carefully spoon the tuna salad into each hollowed cherry tomato, filling them generously.
4. Arrange the stuffed tomatoes on a platter. Serve immediately or refrigerate until ready to serve.

NUTRITION INFORMATION: (APPROXIMATE VALUES PER SERVING): Carbohydrates: 4g | Sodium: 80mg | Fats: 2g | Potassium: 250mg | Sugar: 3g | Cholesterol: 15mg

MINTY PEA AND AVOCADO SPREAD ON WHOLE GRAIN TOAST

This vibrant Minty Pea and Avocado Spread on Whole Grain Toast combines the freshness of mint and peas with the creaminess of the avocado, served on hearty whole-grain toast. It's perfect for a nutritious snack or appetizer, fully compliant with a fatty liver diet.

Prep Time: 10 minutes
Cooking Time: 0 minutes
Complexity: Beginner
Servings: 4
Ingredients: 6

EQUIPMENT NEEDED: Bowl, food processor, toaster

TAGS: High-fiber, Low Sodium, vegetarian, Heart-Healthy, Low Glycemic, Sugar-Free, Whole Foods, low-calorie, Vitamin C rich, Vitamin E rich

INGREDIENT LIST:

- 1 cup (150 g) frozen peas, thawed
- 1 ripe avocado, peeled and pitted
- 1/4 cup (4 g) fresh mint leaves
- 2 tablespoons (30 ml) lemon juice
- Salt and pepper to taste (minimal salt)
- 4 slices whole grain bread

DIRECTIONS:

1. In a food processor, blend the thawed peas, avocado, fresh mint leaves, and lemon juice until smooth. Season with a pinch of salt and pepper to taste, keeping the salt minimal to maintain a low sodium profile.
2. Toast the whole grain bread slices until they are golden and crispy.
3. Spread a generous layer of the pea and avocado mixture onto each slice of toasted bread.
4. Cut each slice into halves or quarters and serve immediately to enjoy the crunch of the toast with the creamy, flavorful spread.

NUTRITION INFORMATION: (APPROXIMATE VALUES PER SERVING): Carbohydrates: 20g | Sodium: 150mg | Fats: 9g | Potassium: 400mg | Sugar: 3g | Cholesterol: 0mg

ROASTED TURMERIC AND CUMIN CAULIFLOWER BITES

Savor the aromatic flavors of these Roasted Turmeric and Cumin Cauliflower Bites, perfect for a healthy snack or appetizer. This dish combines the earthy spice of turmeric and cumin with the natural sweetness of cauliflower, baked to perfection for a delightful crunch.

Prep Time: 10 minutes
Cooking Time: 25 minutes
Complexity: Beginner
Servings: 4
Ingredients: 6

EQUIPMENT NEEDED: Baking sheet, bowl, mixing spoon

TAGS: High-fiber, Low Sodium, vegan, Heart-Healthy, Low Glycemic, Sugar-Free, Whole Foods, gluten-free, low-fat, low-calorie, Vitamin C rich

INGREDIENT LIST:

- 1 large head of cauliflower, cut into bite-sized florets (about 4 cups)
- 2 tablespoons olive oil (30 ml)
- 1 teaspoon ground turmeric (5 ml)
- 1 teaspoon ground cumin (5 ml)
- 1/4 teaspoon salt (1.25 ml) [use a low amount to keep sodium content down]
- Freshly ground black pepper, to taste

DIRECTIONS:

1. Preheat the oven to 400°F (200°C).
2. In a large bowl, combine the cauliflower florets with olive oil, turmeric, cumin, salt, and black pepper. Toss well to ensure each floret is evenly coated with the spices and oil.
3. Spread the cauliflower on a baking sheet in a single layer, making sure they do not overlap to ensure even cooking.
4. Roast in the preheated oven for about 25 minutes or until the cauliflower is tender and the edges are crispy and golden.
5. Remove from the oven and let cool slightly before serving.

NUTRITION INFORMATION: (APPROXIMATE VALUES PER SERVING): Carbohydrates: 10g | Sodium: 150mg | Fats: 8g | Potassium: 470mg | Sugar: 3g | Cholesterol: 0mg

NO-BAKE WALNUT AND DATE ENERGY BALLS

These No-Bake Walnut and Date Energy Balls are a perfect snack for energy boosts and satisfy cravings with natural sweetness and nutty flavors, all while adhering to the fatty liver diet guidelines. Rich in nutrients and fiber, they are a healthy choice any time of the day.

- **Prep Time:** 15 minutes
- **Cooking Time:** 0 minutes
- **Complexity:** Beginner
- **Servings:** 10
- **Ingredients:** 5

EQUIPMENT NEEDED: Food processor, mixing bowl

TAGS: High-fiber, Low Sodium, vegetarian, Heart-Healthy, Low Glycemic, Sugar-Free, Whole Foods, gluten-free, High-protein, low-fat, low-calorie, Vitamin E rich

INGREDIENT LIST:

- 1 cup walnuts (150 g)
- 1 cup pitted dates (175 g)
- 1/4 cup unsweetened cocoa powder (30 g)
- 1 teaspoon vanilla extract (5 ml)
- A pinch of salt

DIRECTIONS:

1. Place the walnuts in a food processor and pulse until finely ground.
2. Add the pitted dates, unsweetened cocoa powder, vanilla extract, and a pinch of salt to the food processor. Pulse until the mixture becomes sticky and clumps together.
3. Remove the mixture from the food processor and roll it into small balls, about the size of a tablespoon each.
4. Place the energy balls on a plate or baking sheet lined with parchment paper. Refrigerate for at least 30 minutes to set, making them easier to handle and more cohesive.
5. Store in an airtight container in the refrigerator for up to a week or freeze for longer storage.

NUTRITION INFORMATION: (APPROXIMATE VALUES PER SERVING): Carbohydrates: 15g | Sodium: 10mg | Fats: 8g | Potassium: 200mg | Sugar: 12g | Cholesterol: 0mg

AVOCADO AND LIME FROZEN YOGURT

This refreshing Avocado and Lime Frozen Yogurt combines creamy textures and zesty flavors, making it an ideal treat for those following a fatty liver diet. Packed with healthy fats and low in sugar, it's a delightful way to satisfy your sweet tooth without straying from dietary guidelines.

- **Prep Time:** 10 minutes
- **Cooking Time:** 0 minutes
- **Complexity:** Beginner
- **Servings:** 4
- **Ingredients:** 5

EQUIPMENT NEEDED: Food processor, mixing bowl, freezer-safe container

TAGS: Low Sodium, High-fiber, vegetarian, gluten-free, High-protein, low-fat, Heart-Healthy, Whole Foods, Low Glycemic, Sugar-Free, low-calorie, Vitamin C rich

INGREDIENT LIST:

- 2 ripe avocados, peeled and pitted (200 g each)
- 2 cups plain low-fat Greek yogurt (480 ml)
- 1/4 cup freshly squeezed lime juice (60 ml)
- 2 tablespoons honey (optional, for a touch of sweetness) (30 ml)
- Zest of 1 lime

DIRECTIONS:

1. In a food processor, blend the avocados, Greek yogurt, lime juice, honey (if using), and lime zest until smooth.
2. Taste the mixture and adjust the sweetness if necessary.
3. Pour the mixture into a freezer-safe container and smooth the top with a spatula.
4. Cover and freeze for at least 4 hours, stirring every hour if possible, to help break up ice crystals and improve the texture.
5. Once set, scoop and serve immediately, or store in the freezer in an airtight container for up to 1 month.

NUTRITION INFORMATION (APPROXIMATE VALUES PER SERVING): Carbohydrates: 18g | Sodium: 60mg | Fats: 15g | Potassium: 708mg | Sugar: 6g (natural sugars from the fruit, not including optional honey) | Cholesterol: 10mg

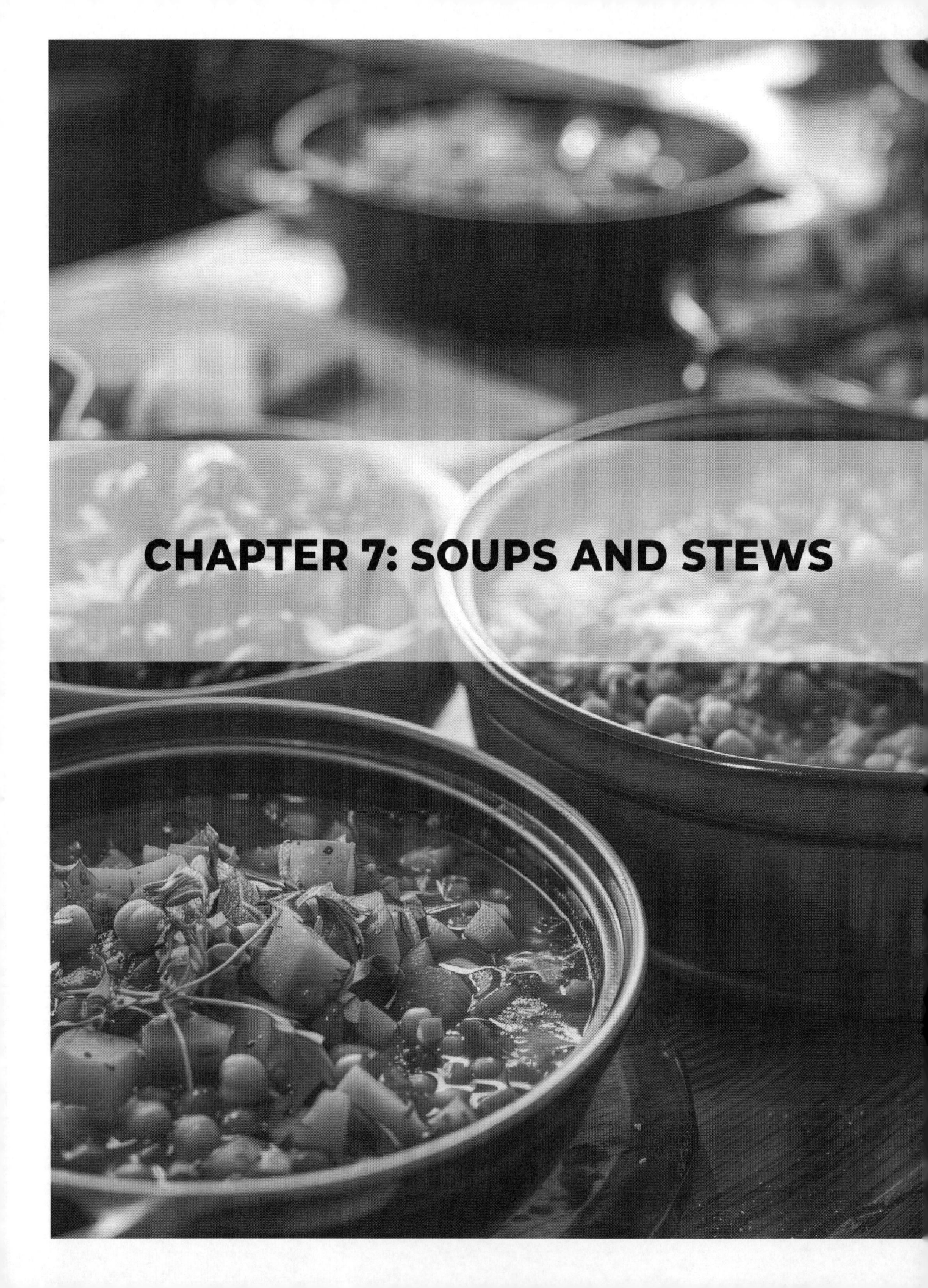

CHAPTER 7: SOUPS AND STEWS

COMFORTING AND HEALING SOUPS AND STEWS

COD AND PARSNIP STEW

This Cod and Parsnip Stew is a hearty and healthy dish perfect for a fatty liver diet. Rich in omega-3 fatty acids, high in fiber, and low in sodium, this stew provides a nourishing meal that supports liver health while satisfying your taste buds.

Prep Time: 15 minutes | **Cooking Time:** 30 minutes | **Complexity:** Beginner | **Servings:** 4 | **Ingredients:** 8

EQUIPMENT NEEDED: Large pot, cutting board, knife

TAGS: High Protein, High Fiber, Low Sodium, Heart-Healthy, Whole Foods, Low Glycemic, Low Fat, Vitamin A rich, Vitamin C rich, gluten-free, dairy-free

INGREDIENT LIST:

- 1 lb (450 g) cod fillets, cut into chunks, 3 large parsnips, peeled and diced (about 3 cups)
- 1 onion, finely chopped
- 2 cloves garlic, minced
- 4 cups low-sodium vegetable broth (960 ml)
- 1 teaspoon turmeric powder
- 1 teaspoon cumin powder, Fresh parsley, chopped, for garnish
- Salt and pepper to taste (optional, mindful of sodium intake)

DIRECTIONS:

1. In a large pot, sauté the onion and garlic over medium heat until translucent, about 5 minutes. Add the parsnips to the pot and cook for another 5 minutes, stirring occasionally.
2. Sprinkle in the turmeric and cumin, and stir to coat the vegetables evenly.
3. Pour in the vegetable broth and bring the mixture to a boil. Once boiling, reduce the heat to low and simmer for 15 minutes or until the parsnips are tender.
4. Add the cod chunks to the pot, and simmer for an additional 10 minutes, or until the fish is cooked through and flakes easily.
5. Season with salt and pepper if desired, keeping sodium guidelines in mind. Garnish with fresh parsley before serving.

NUTRITION INFORMATION: (APPROXIMATE VALUES PER SERVING): Carbohydrates: 28g | Sodium: 300mg | Fats: 3g | Potassium: 850mg | Sugar: 9g | Cholesterol: 60mg

BLACK BEAN AND BUTTERNUT SQUASH STEW

This hearty Black Bean and Butternut Squash Stew is a delightful blend of rich flavors and textures, perfect for promoting liver health. Loaded with fiber, plant-based protein, and healthy fats, it's a satisfying dish that adheres to the fatty liver diet guidelines.

Prep Time: 20 minutes | **Cooking Time:** 45 minutes | **Complexity:** Beginner | **Servings:** 6 | **Ingredients:** 12

EQUIPMENT NEEDED: Large pot, knife, cutting board

TAGS: Vegan, High Fiber, Low Sodium, Low Fat, Heart-Healthy, Whole Foods, Low Glycemic, Sugar-Free, High Protein, Vitamin A rich, Vitamin C rich, gluten-free, dairy-free

INGREDIENT LIST:

- 1 butternut squash, peeled and cubed (about 3 cups)
- 2 cans (15 oz each) black beans, drained and rinsed, 1 large onion, chopped
- 3 cloves garlic, minced
- 1 red bell pepper, diced
- 1 tablespoon olive oil, 4 cups low-sodium vegetable broth (950 ml), 2 teaspoons ground cumin
- 1 teaspoon smoked paprika
- 1/2 teaspoon chili powder
- Salt and pepper to taste (optional; keep sodium intake in mind)
- Fresh cilantro, chopped for garnish

DIRECTIONS:

1. Heat olive oil in a large pot over medium heat. Add onions and garlic, and sauté until onions are translucent, about 5 minutes.
2. Add red bell pepper and cubed butternut squash to the pot, stir to combine, and cook for another 5 minutes.
3. Stir in ground cumin, smoked paprika, and chili powder, and cook for 1 minute until fragrant.
4. Pour in the vegetable broth and bring to a boil. Once boiling, reduce heat to a simmer and cook for 25 minutes or until the squash is tender.
5. Add the black beans to the pot and continue to simmer for an additional 15 minutes. Season with salt and pepper if desired, keeping in mind the dietary sodium restrictions.
6. Serve hot, garnished with fresh cilantro.

NUTRITION INFORMATION: (APPROXIMATE VALUES PER SERVING): Carbohydrates: 45g | Sodium: 300mg | Fats: 3g | Potassium: 600mg | Sugar: 7g | Cholesterol: 0mg

PUMPKIN AND CHICKPEA STEW

This Pumpkin and Chickpea Stew is a comforting, nutrient-dense dish perfect for a fatty liver diet. Packed with fiber, low in fat, and rich in plant-based proteins, it supports liver health while being hearty and delicious.

Prep Time: 15 minutes
Cooking Time: 40 minutes
Complexity: Beginner
Servings: 4
Ingredients: 10

EQUIPMENT NEEDED: Large pot, knife, cutting board

TAGS: Vegan, High Fiber, Low Sodium, Low Fat, Heart-Healthy, Whole Foods, Low Glycemic, Sugar-Free, High Protein, Vitamin A rich, Vitamin C rich, gluten-free, dairy-free

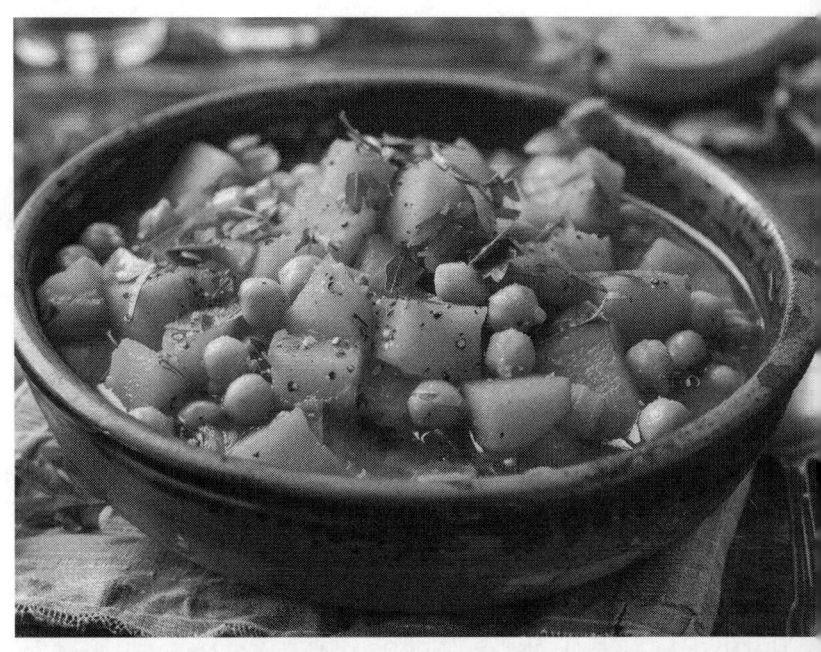

INGREDIENT LIST:

- 2 cups pumpkin, peeled and cubed (about 300 g)
- 1 can (15 oz or 425 g) chickpeas, drained and rinsed
- 1 large onion, diced
- 2 cloves garlic, minced
- 1 red bell pepper, diced
- 4 cups low-sodium vegetable broth (960 ml)
- 2 teaspoons cumin powder
- 1 teaspoon smoked paprika
- 1 tablespoon olive oil
- Salt and pepper to taste (optional, mindful of sodium intake)
- Fresh cilantro, chopped for garnish

DIRECTIONS:

1. Heat the olive oil in a large pot over medium heat. Add the onion and garlic, sautéing until the onion becomes translucent, about 5 minutes.
2. Add the red bell pepper and pumpkin to the pot and cook for another 5 minutes, stirring occasionally.
3. Stir in the cumin and smoked paprika, cooking for another minute until fragrant.
4. Pour in the vegetable broth, bring the mixture to a boil, then reduce the heat and simmer for 20 minutes or until the pumpkin is tender.
5. Add the chickpeas to the pot and continue to simmer for an additional 10 minutes.
6. Season with salt and pepper if desired, keeping sodium guidelines in mind.
7. Serve the stew garnished with fresh cilantro.

NUTRITION INFORMATION: (APPROXIMATE VALUES PER SERVING): Carbohydrates: 45g | Sodium: 300mg | Fats: 5g | Potassium: 600mg | Sugar: 12g | Cholesterol: 0mg

TURKEY AND QUINOA STEW

A hearty, nourishing stew perfect for supporting liver health with lean protein and high-fiber ingredients, suitable for a cozy family dinner.

- **Prep Time:** 20 minutes
- **Cooking Time:** 40 minutes
- **Complexity:** Beginner
- **Servings:** 4
- **Ingredients:** 10

EQUIPMENT NEEDED: arge pot, chopping board, knife, measuring cups, measuring spoons
TAGS: High-protein, High-fiber, Low Sodium, Heart-Healthy, Whole Foods, Low Glycemic

INGREDIENT LIST:

- 1 lb (450 g) lean ground turkey
- 1 cup (190 g) quinoa, rinsed
- 1 large carrot, diced (about 1 cup or 130 g)
- 2 stalks celery, diced (about 1 cup or 100 g)
- 1 medium onion, chopped (about 1 cup or 150 g), 3 cloves garlic, minced
- 1 teaspoon (5 ml) olive oil
- 4 cups (950 ml) low-sodium vegetable broth, 1 teaspoon (5 ml) dried thyme
- Salt and pepper to taste (use minimal salt)

DIRECTIONS:

1. Heat the olive oil in a large pot over medium heat. Add the chopped onions, carrots, celery, and minced garlic, sautéing until the onions become translucent.
2. Add the ground turkey to the pot and cook until it is browned, breaking it up as it cooks.
3. Stir in the rinsed quinoa, dried thyme, and low-sodium vegetable broth. Bring the mixture to a boil.
4. Reduce the heat to a simmer, cover the pot, and let it cook for about 30 minutes, or until the quinoa is fully cooked and the vegetables are tender.
5. Season with minimal salt and pepper to taste. Serve hot.

NUTRITION INFORMATION: (APPROXIMATE VALUES PER SERVING): Calories: 330 | Protein: 26g | carbohydrates: 36g | Fats: 8g | Sodium: 200 mg | Sugar: 4g | Cholesterol: 55 mg

---

SPECIAL SECTION: QUICK & EASY ONE-POT WONDERS

MUSHROOM AND BARLEY SOUP

This Mushroom and Barley Soup is a warm, comforting dish packed with fiber and essential nutrients, ideal for those adhering to a fatty liver diet.

- **Prep Time:** 15 minutes
- **Cooking Time:** 60 minutes
- **Complexity:** Beginner
- **Servings:** 6
- **Ingredients:** 9

EQUIPMENT NEEDED: large pot, knife, cutting board, measuring cups, measuring spoons
TAGS: High-fiber, Whole Foods, Low Glycemic, Heart-Healthy, Vegetarian, Low Sodium, Low Fat

INGREDIENT LIST:

- 1 tablespoon (15 ml) olive oil
- 1 large onion, diced (about 1 cup or 150 g)
- 2 garlic cloves, minced
- 1 pound (450 g) fresh mushrooms, sliced (such as cremini or button)
- 3/4 cup (120 g) pearl barley, rinsed
- 6 cups (1.4 liters) low-sodium vegetable broth
- 2 carrots, peeled and diced (about 1 cup or 130 g)
- 2 celery stalks, diced (about 1 cup or 100 g)
- Fresh herbs (such as parsley or thyme) for garnish, chopped

DIRECTIONS:

1. Heat the olive oil in a large pot over medium heat. Add the diced onion and minced garlic, cooking until the onion is translucent.
2. Add the sliced mushrooms to the pot and sauté until they begin to brown and release their juices, about 8 minutes.
3. Stir in the pearl barley, then pour in the low-sodium vegetable broth. Bring to a boil.
4. Once boiling, reduce the heat to a simmer, add the diced carrots and celery, and cover the pot. Let it simmer for about 50 minutes or until the barley is tender.
5. Serve the soup garnished with fresh herbs like parsley or thyme.

NUTRITION INFORMATION: (APPROXIMATE VALUES PER SERVING): Calories: 200 | Protein: 6g | carbohydrates: 40g | Fats: 3g | Sodium: 120 mg | Sugar: 5g | Cholesterol: 0 mg

VEGETABLE AND TEMPEH STEW

This Vegetable and Tempeh Stew is a nutrient-rich, plant-based meal perfect for supporting liver health. Featuring a variety of vegetables and tempeh as a lean protein source, this stew is hearty, flavorful, and aligns with the fatty liver diet guidelines.

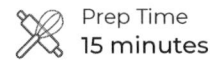

Prep Time: 15 minutes
Cooking Time: 30 minutes
Complexity: Beginner
Servings: 4
Ingredients: 12

EQUIPMENT NEEDED: Large pot, knife, cutting board

TAGS: Vegan, High Fiber, Low Sodium, Low Fat, Heart-Healthy, Whole Foods, Low Glycemic, Sugar-Free, High Protein, Vitamin C rich, gluten-free, dairy-free

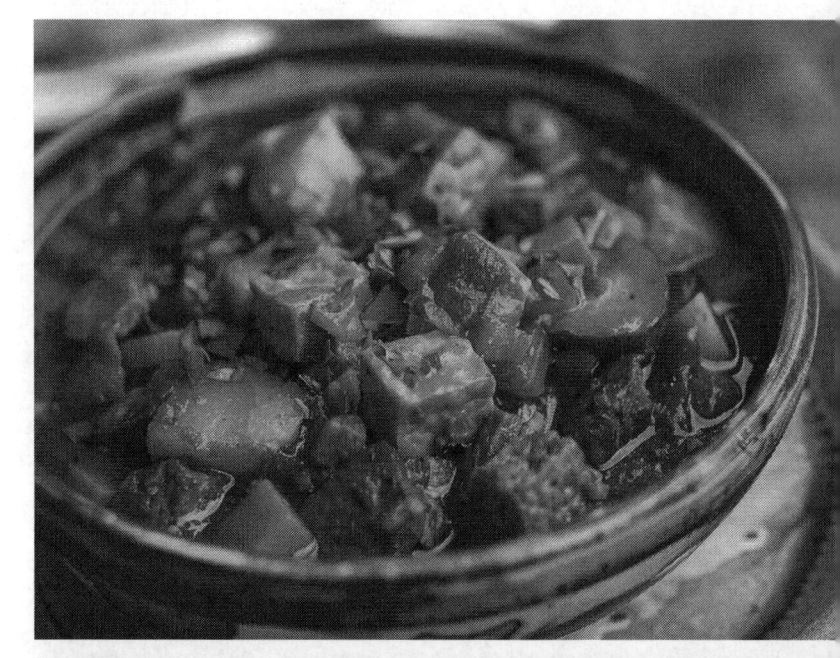

INGREDIENT LIST:

- 8 oz tempeh, cubed (about 225 g)
- 1 tablespoon olive oil
- 1 large onion, chopped
- 2 cloves garlic, minced
- 2 carrots, peeled and diced
- 2 stalks celery, chopped
- 1 red bell pepper, chopped
- 1 zucchini, chopped
- 3 cups vegetable broth (about 700 ml)
- 1 can (14.5 oz) diced tomatoes, no salt added
- 1 teaspoon dried thyme
- Salt and pepper to taste (optional, mindful of sodium intake)
- Fresh parsley, chopped for garnish

DIRECTIONS:

1. Heat olive oil in a large pot over medium heat. Add onion and garlic, and sauté until onions are translucent, about 5 minutes.
2. Add carrots, celery, bell pepper, and zucchini to the pot. Cook for another 5 minutes, stirring occasionally.
3. Incorporate the cubed tempeh and cook for 5 minutes, allowing the tempeh to brown slightly.
4. Pour in the vegetable broth and add the diced tomatoes and dried thyme. Bring the mixture to a boil.
5. Once boiling, reduce the heat and let simmer for 20 minutes or until the vegetables are tender.
6. Season with salt and pepper if desired, keeping sodium intake in mind.
7. Serve hot, garnished with fresh parsley.

NUTRITION INFORMATION: (APPROXIMATE VALUES PER SERVING): Carbohydrates: 26g | Sodium: 280mg | Fats: 8g | Potassium: 600mg | Sugar: 10g | Cholesterol: 0mg

KALE AND WHITE BEAN SOUP

This nutrient-dense soup combines the heartiness of white beans with the robust flavors of kale, making it a perfect addition to a fatty liver diet plan.

Prep Time: 15 minutes | **Cooking Time:** 30 minutes | **Complexity:** Beginner | **Servings:** 6 | **Ingredients:** 8

EQUIPMENT NEEDED: large pot, knife, cutting board, measuring cups, measuring spoons

TAGS: High-fiber, Low Sodium, Heart-Healthy, Whole Foods, Low Glycemic, Vegetarian, Low Fat, High-protein, Vitamin A rich, Vitamin C rich

INGREDIENT LIST:

- 1 tablespoon (15 ml) olive oil
- 1 large onion, chopped (about 1 cup or 150 g), 2 garlic cloves, minced, 4 cups (1 liter) low-sodium vegetable broth
- 1 can (15 ounces or 425 g) white beans, drained and rinsed
- 4 cups (roughly 200 g) chopped kale, stems removed
- 2 carrots, peeled and diced (about 1 cup or 130 g)
- 1 teaspoon (5 ml) dried thyme
- Salt and pepper to taste (use minimal salt)

DIRECTIONS:

1. Heat the olive oil in a large pot over medium heat. Add the chopped onion and minced garlic and sauté until the onions are translucent.
2. Add the diced carrots to the pot, cooking for about 5 minutes until they start to soften.
3. Pour in the low-sodium vegetable broth and bring the mixture to a boil.
4. Reduce the heat to a simmer and add the white beans, chopped kale, and dried thyme. Cook for another 15-20 minutes, until the kale is tender and the flavors are well blended.
5. Season with minimal salt and pepper to taste. Serve hot.

NUTRITION INFORMATION: (APPROXIMATE VALUES PER SERVING): Calories: 180 | Protein: 10g | carbohydrates: 30g | Fats: 3g | Sodium: 150 mg | Sugar: 3g | Cholesterol: 0 mg

SPICY TOMATO AND LENTIL SOUP

This Spicy Tomato and Lentil Soup is a vibrant, flavor-packed dish that supports liver health with its high fiber and protein content, perfect for a wholesome meal.

Prep Time: 10 minutes | **Cooking Time:** 45 minutes | **Complexity:** Beginner | **Servings:** 6 | **Ingredients:** 10

EQUIPMENT NEEDED: large pot, knife, cutting board, measuring cups, measuring spoons

TAGS: High-fiber, Low Sodium, Heart-Healthy, Whole Foods, Low Glycemic, Vegan, High-protein, Low Fat, Vitamin C rich

INGREDIENT LIST:

- 1 tablespoon (15 ml) olive oil
- 1 large onion, chopped (about 1 cup or 150 g)
- 2 cloves garlic, minced
- 1 teaspoon (5 ml) crushed red pepper flakes (adjust based on spice preference)
- 1 cup (192 g) dried lentils, rinsed
- 1 can (28 ounces or 794 g) no-salt-added diced tomatoes
- 6 cups (1.4 liters) low-sodium vegetable broth
- 1 teaspoon (5 ml) ground cumin
- 1 teaspoon (5 ml) smoked paprika
- 2 medium carrots, diced (about 1 cup or 130 g)

DIRECTIONS:

1. Heat the olive oil in a large pot over medium heat. Add the chopped onion and minced garlic, sautéing until the onion is translucent.
2. Stir in the crushed red pepper flakes, ground cumin, and smoked paprika, cooking for about 1 minute to release the flavors.
3. Add the dried lentils, diced tomatoes, and diced carrots to the pot, mixing well.
4. Pour in the low-sodium vegetable broth and bring the mixture to a boil.
5. Reduce the heat to a simmer and cook, covered, for about 35-40 minutes, or until the lentils are tender and the soup has thickened.
6. Adjust the seasoning with salt and more red pepper flakes if desired. Serve hot.

NUTRITION INFORMATION: (APPROXIMATE VALUES PER SERVING): Calories: 220 | Protein: 14g | carbohydrates: 38g | Fats: 3g | Sodium: 150 mg | Sugar: 6g | Cholesterol: 0 mg

CREAMY AVOCADO AND CUCUMBER SOUP

This refreshing and creamy soup combines avocado and cucumber for a deliciously smooth texture, rich in healthy fats, and perfect for a light meal.

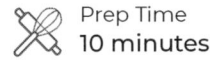

Prep Time: 10 minutes
Cooking Time: 0 minutes
Complexity: Beginner
Servings: 4
Ingredients: 7

EQUIPMENT NEEDED: blender, measuring cups, measuring spoons, knife, cutting board

TAGS: Heart-Healthy, Whole Foods, Vegan, Low Glycemic, Low Sodium, Low Fat, High-fiber, Vitamin C rich, Vitamin E rich

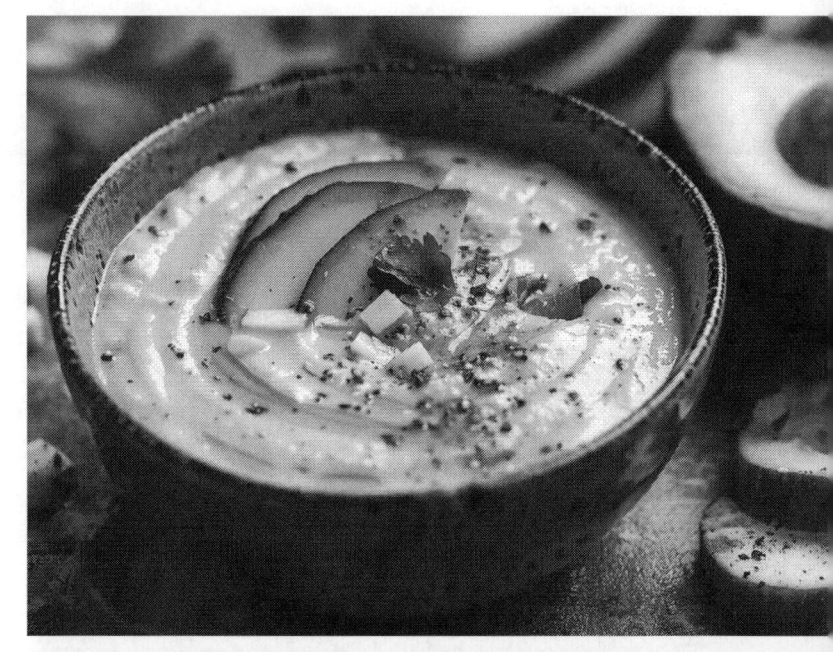

INGREDIENT LIST:

- 2 ripe avocados, peeled and pitted
- 1 large cucumber, peeled and chopped
- 2 cups (480 ml) cold water
- Juice of 1 lemon (about 2 tablespoons or 30 ml)
- 1 clove garlic, minced
- Salt to taste (minimal)
- Fresh herbs (such as dill or parsley), for garnish

DIRECTIONS:

1. Combine the peeled and pitted avocados, chopped cucumber, cold water, lemon juice, and minced garlic in a blender.
2. Blend until the mixture is completely smooth. If the soup is too thick, add a little more water until the desired consistency is reached.
3. Taste and season with a minimal amount of salt.
4. Chill the soup in the refrigerator for at least 30 minutes before serving.
5. Serve cold, garnished with fresh herbs like dill or parsley.

NUTRITION INFORMATION: (APPROXIMATE VALUES PER SERVING): Calories: 160 | Protein: 2g | carbohydrates: 12g | Fats: 12g | Sodium: 10 mg | Potassium: 487 mg | Sugar: 1g | Cholesterol: 0 mg

CHAPTER 8: HEALTHY MEAT DISHES

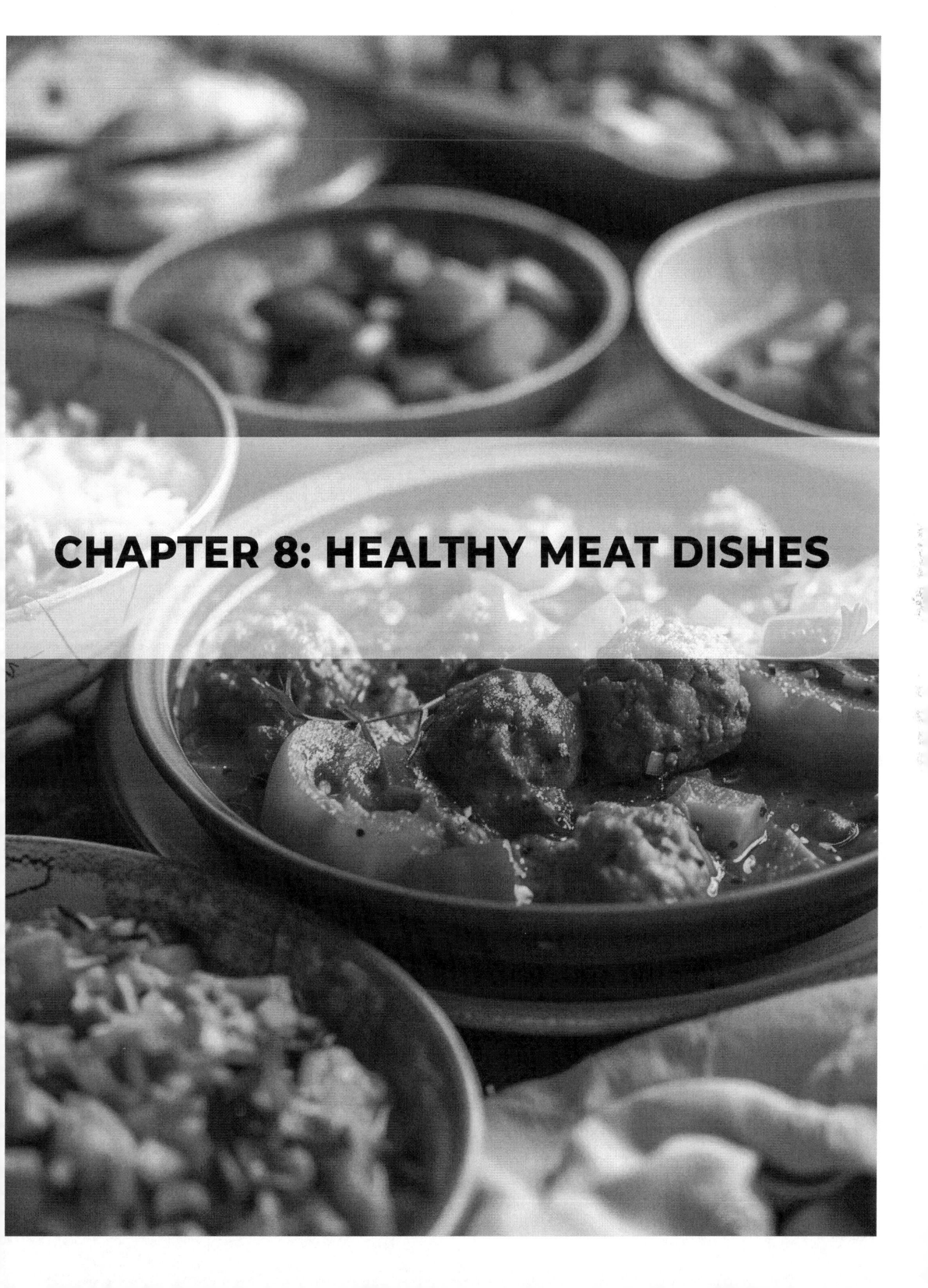

MOROCCAN SPICED CHICKEN STEW WITH APRICOTS

This Moroccan-inspired chicken stew combines sweet apricots with aromatic spices, providing a hearty dish rich in protein and flavors while adhering to fatty liver diet guidelines.

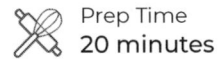

Prep Time 20 minutes | **Cooking Time** 40 minutes | **Complexity** Intermediate | **Servings** 4 | **Ingredients** 12

EQUIPMENT NEEDED: large pot, knife, cutting board, measuring spoons, measuring cups

TAGS: High-protein, Low Sodium, Heart-Healthy, Whole Foods, Low Glycemic, Low Fat, High-fiber, Vitamin A rich

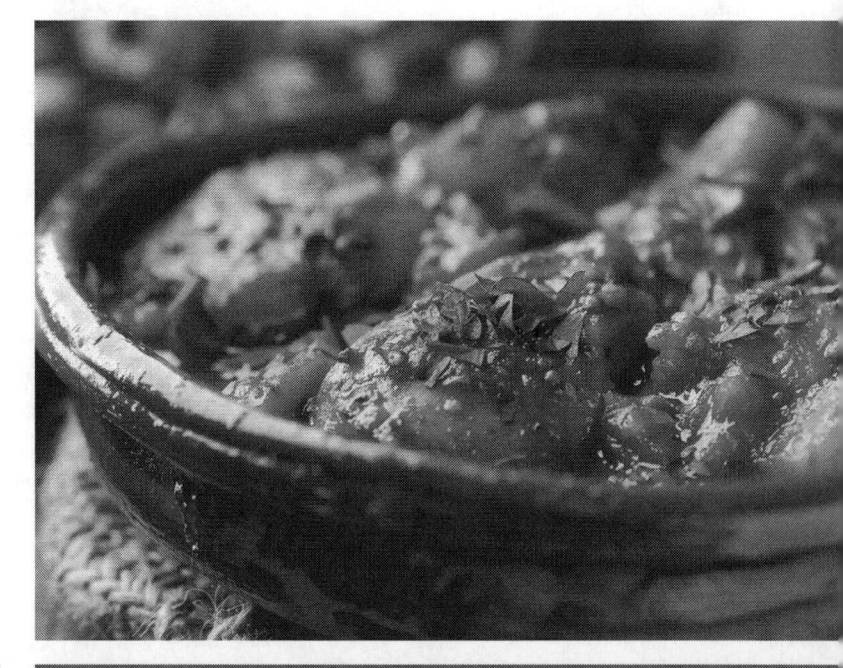

INGREDIENT LIST:

- 1 tablespoon (15 ml) olive oil
- 1 pound (450 g) boneless, skinless chicken thighs, trimmed and cut into pieces
- 1 large onion, chopped (about 1 cup or 150 g)
- 3 cloves garlic, minced
- 1 tablespoon (15 ml) ground cumin
- 1 teaspoon (5 ml) ground cinnamon
- 1/2 teaspoon (2.5 ml) ground turmeric
- 1/2 teaspoon (2.5 ml) ground ginger
- 2 cups (480 ml) low-sodium chicken broth
- 1/2 cup (about 80 g) dried apricots, chopped
- 1 can (14.5 ounces or 411 g) no-salt-added diced tomatoes
- 1 can (15 ounces or 425 g) chickpeas, rinsed and drained

DIRECTIONS:

1. Heat the olive oil in a large pot over medium-high heat. Add the chicken pieces and cook until browned on all sides.
2. Add the chopped onion and minced garlic to the pot with the chicken and sauté until the onions are translucent.
3. Stir in the cumin, cinnamon, turmeric, and ginger, cooking for about 1 minute until fragrant.
4. Pour in the low-sodium chicken broth, and add the chopped dried apricots and diced tomatoes. Bring to a boil.
5. Reduce the heat to low, cover, and simmer for 30 minutes.
6. Stir in the chickpeas and continue to simmer for an additional 10 minutes.
7. Adjust seasoning with a minimal amount of salt, if necessary, and pepper to taste before serving.

NUTRITION INFORMATION: (APPROXIMATE VALUES PER SERVING): Calories: 350 | Protein: 28g | carbohydrates: 35g | Fats: 12g | Sodium: 300 mg | Potassium: 800 mg | Sugar: 15g | Cholesterol: 80 mg

ASIAN-STYLE TURKEY MEATBALLS WITH VEGETABLE STIR FRY

This dish combines the lean protein of turkey with a vibrant mix of vegetables, all flavored with Asian-inspired spices, making it a wholesome meal perfect for supporting liver health.

- **Prep Time:** 20 minutes
- **Cooking Time:** 30 minutes
- **Complexity:** Intermediate
- **Servings:** 4
- **Ingredients:** 14

EQUIPMENT NEEDED: mixing bowl, skillet, spoon, knife, cutting board
TAGS: High-protein, Low Sodium, Heart-Healthy, Whole Foods, Low Glycemic, Low Fat, High-fiber, Vitamin C rich

INGREDIENT LIST:

- 1 pound (450 g) ground turkey (lean), 1 large egg, beaten, 2 cloves garlic, minced
- 1 inch (2.5 cm) fresh ginger, grated
- 2 green onions, finely chopped
- 2 tablespoons (30 ml) low-sodium soy sauce, 1 tablespoon (15 ml) sesame oil
- 1 teaspoon (5 ml) Sriracha sauce (adjust to taste), 1/2 cup (50 g) breadcrumbs (whole grain, if possible)
- 2 cups (200 g) broccoli florets
- 1 red bell pepper, sliced
- 1 carrot, julienned
- 1 zucchini, sliced
- 1 tablespoon (15 ml) olive oil

DIRECTIONS:

1. In a bowl, combine the ground turkey, beaten egg, half of the minced garlic, ginger, green onions, 1 tablespoon of soy sauce, breadcrumbs, and Sriracha sauce. Mix well.
2. Form the mixture into small meatballs about 1 inch in diameter. Heat the sesame oil in a skillet over medium heat and cook the meatballs until browned and cooked through, about 10-15 minutes, turning occasionally.
3. In another skillet, heat the olive oil over medium heat. Add the remaining garlic, broccoli, red bell pepper, carrot, and zucchini. Stir-fry until the vegetables are tender-crisp, about 8-10 minutes.
4. Drizzle the remaining soy sauce over the vegetables during the last few minutes of cooking.
5. Serve the meatballs with the vegetable stir-fry on the side or mixed together.

NUTRITION INFORMATION: (APPROXIMATE VALUES PER SERVING): Calories: 350 | Protein: 28g | carbohydrates: 22g | Fats: 18g | Sodium: 400 mg | Potassium: 650 mg | Sugar: 6g | Cholesterol: 80 mg

STUFFED PEPPERS WITH GROUND CHICKEN AND BROWN RICE

This dish combines the nutritional benefits of colorful bell peppers stuffed with lean ground chicken and fiber-rich brown rice seasoned with herbs for a wholesome and satisfying meal.

- **Prep Time:** 15 minutes
- **Cooking Time:** 45 minutes
- **Complexity:** Beginner
- **Servings:** 4
- **Ingredients:** 9

EQUIPMENT NEEDED: skillet, baking dish, knife, cutting board, mixing bowl, spoon
TAGS: High-protein, High-fiber, Low Sodium, Heart-Healthy, Whole Foods, Low Glycemic, Low Fat, Vitamin C rich

INGREDIENT LIST:

- 4 large bell peppers, tops cut off and seeds removed, 1 tablespoon (15 ml) olive oil
- 1 onion, finely chopped
- 2 cloves garlic, minced
- 1 pound (450 g) ground chicken (lean)
- 1 cup (185 g) cooked brown rice
- 1 can (15 ounces or 425 g) diced tomatoes, no salt added, drained
- 1 teaspoon (5 ml) dried basil
- 1 teaspoon (5 ml) dried oregano
- Salt and pepper to taste (use minimal salt)

DIRECTIONS:

1. Preheat the oven to 375°F (190°C). In a skillet, heat the olive oil over medium heat. Add the onion and garlic, sautéing until the onion becomes translucent.
2. Add the ground chicken to the skillet, breaking it up with a spoon. Cook until the chicken is thoroughly cooked and no longer pink. Stir in the cooked brown rice, drained tomatoes, basil, oregano, and season with minimal salt and pepper. Cook together for an additional 5 minutes, allowing the flavors to blend.
3. Spoon the chicken and rice mixture into the hollowed-out bell peppers. Place the stuffed peppers in a baking dish and cover with foil. Bake in the preheated oven for 30-35 minutes until the peppers are tender.
4. Remove the foil and bake for an additional 10 minutes to lightly brown the tops.

NUTRITION INFORMATION: (APPROXIMATE VALUES PER SERVING): Calories: 290 | Protein: 26g | carbohydrates: 28g | Fats: 9g | Sodium: 150 mg | Potassium: 650 mg | Sugar: 6g | Cholesterol: 65 mg

SLOW-COOKED TURKEY CHILI WITH SWEET POTATOES

This hearty chili uses lean ground turkey and sweet potatoes, enriched with spices for a flavorful and nutritious dish that fits perfectly within a fatty liver diet.

Prep Time: 15 minutes
Cooking Time: 4 or 8 hours
Complexity: Beginner
Servings: 6
Ingredients: 11

EQUIPMENT NEEDED: slow cooker, skillet, knife, cutting board, measuring cups, measuring spoons
TAGS: High-protein, High-fiber, Low Sodium, Heart-Healthy, Whole Foods, Low Glycemic, Low Fat, Vitamin A rich

INGREDIENT LIST:

- 1 tablespoon (15 ml) olive oil
- 1 large onion, chopped (about 1 cup or 150 g), 2 cups (480 ml) low-sodium chicken broth, 2 cloves garlic, minced, 1 pound (450 g) ground turkey, lean
- 2 large sweet potatoes, peeled & cubed (about 3 cups or 400 g)
- 1 can (15 ounces or 425 g) black beans, rinsed and drained
- 1 can (28 ounces or 794 g) diced tomatoes, no salt added
- 2 tablespoons (30 ml) chili powder
- 1 teaspoon (5 ml) ground cumin
- Salt and pepper to taste (use minimal salt)

DIRECTIONS:

1. Heat olive oil in a skillet over medium heat. Add chopped onion and garlic, and sauté until onion is translucent.
2. Add ground turkey to the skillet. Cook until browned and crumbled. Drain any excess fat.
3. Transfer the browned turkey, onions, and garlic to the slow cooker.
4. Add cubed sweet potatoes, black beans, diced tomatoes, chicken broth, chili powder, and cumin to the slow cooker. Stir to combine all ingredients.
5. Set the slow cooker to low and cook for 8 hours or high for 4 hours, until sweet potatoes are tender and flavors have melded together.
6. Season with minimal salt and pepper to taste before serving.

NUTRITION INFORMATION: (APPROXIMATE VALUES PER SERVING): Calories: 320 | Protein: 24g | carbohydrates: 45g | Fats: 6g | Sodium: 250 mg | Potassium: 850 mg | Sugar: 8g | Cholesterol: 55 mg

BALSAMIC GLAZED DUCK BREAST WITH PEAR CHUTNEY

This recipe features lean duck breast in a balsamic glaze, paired with fresh, homemade pear chutney, perfectly aligning with a fatty liver diet by prioritizing low-fat, high-protein, and whole foods ingredients.

Prep Time: 20 minutes
Cooking Time: 30 minutes
Complexity: Intermediate
Servings: 4
Ingredients: 12

EQUIPMENT NEEDED: skillet, mixing bowl, cutting board, knife, measuring cups, measuring spoons
TAGS: High-protein, Whole Foods, Heart-Healthy, Low Sodium, High-fiber, Low-fat

INGREDIENT LIST:

- 4 boneless duck breasts (about 6 ounces each) (170 g each), 1/2 cup water (120 ml)
- 1 tablespoon olive oil (15 ml), 2 pears, peeled and diced (approx. 150 g each)
- 1 small red onion, finely chopped (approx. 70 g), 1/4 cup balsamic vinegar (60 ml)
- 2 tablespoons honey (30 ml), 1 teaspoon freshly grated ginger (5 g)
- 1/4 teaspoon ground cinnamon (1.25 ml)
- 1/4 cup dried cranberries (30 g)
- Salt to taste (minimal)
- Freshly ground black pepper to taste

DIRECTIONS:

1. Preheat the skillet over medium heat. Rub duck breasts with olive oil, salt, and pepper.
2. Place duck breasts skin side down in the skillet and cook for 8 minutes until the skin is crisp. Flip and cook for another 7-10 minutes or until desired doneness. Remove from skillet and let rest.
3. In the same skillet, add onions and cook until translucent. Add diced pears, ginger, cinnamon, and cranberries. Cook for 5 minutes until pears are soft.
4. Pour in balsamic vinegar, honey, and water. Stir well and simmer until the mixture thickens into a chutney, about 10 minutes. Slice the duck breasts and serve with the warm pear chutney.

NUTRITION INFORMATION: (APPROXIMATE VALUES PER SERVING): Calories: 355 | Protein: 24g | Carbohydrates: 27g | Sodium: 85mg | Fats: 15g | Potassium: 500mg | Sugar: 22g | Cholesterol: 95mg

BEEF AND VEGETABLE KEBABS WITH TZATZIKI

These flavorful kebabs combine lean beef and a variety of vegetables, served with a cooling tzatziki sauce. They are perfect for a healthy meal that supports liver function while being delicious and satisfying.

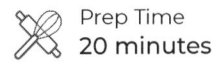

Prep Time: 20 minutes
Cooking Time: 10 minutes
Complexity: Beginner
Servings: 4
Ingredients: 12

EQUIPMENT NEEDED: grill or grill pan, mixing bowls, skewers, knife, cutting board

TAGS: High-protein, Low Sodium, Heart-Healthy, Whole Foods, Low Glycemic, Low Fat, High-fiber, Vitamin A rich

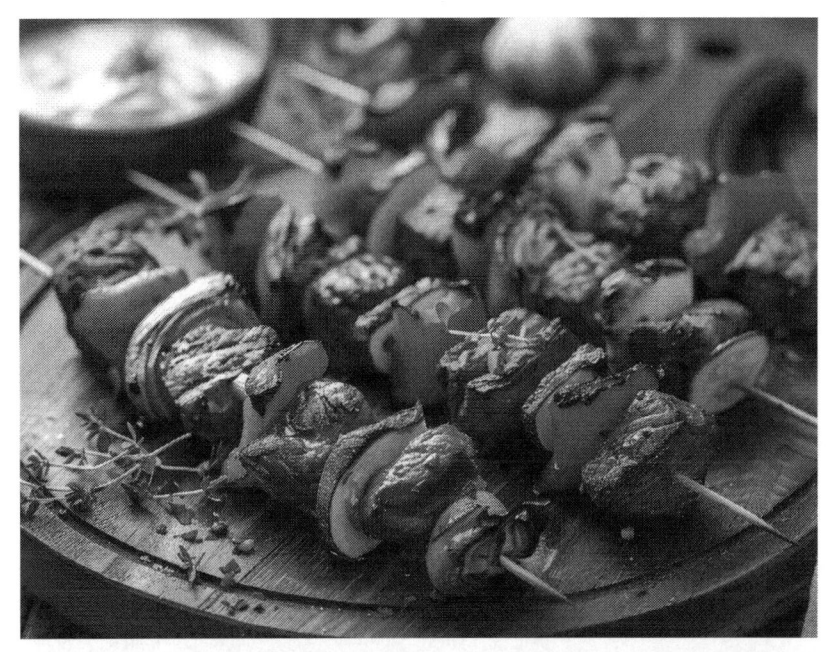

INGREDIENT LIST:

- 1 pound (450 g) lean beef sirloin, cut into 1-inch cubes
- 2 bell peppers (any color), cut into 1-inch pieces
- 1 zucchini, sliced into 1/2-inch thick rounds
- 1 red onion, cut into chunks
- 2 tablespoons (30 ml) olive oil
- 1 teaspoon (5 ml) dried oregano
- 1 teaspoon (5 ml) garlic powder
- Salt and pepper to taste (minimal salt)

For the Tzatziki:

- 1 cup (245 g) plain low-fat Greek yogurt
- 1 small cucumber, finely grated and drained
- 2 cloves garlic, minced
- 1 tablespoon (15 ml) fresh lemon juice
- 1 tablespoon (15 ml) chopped fresh dill

DIRECTIONS:

1. Preheat the grill to medium-high heat. If using wooden skewers, soak them in water for at least 30 minutes to prevent burning.
2. In a large bowl, toss the beef cubes with olive oil, oregano, garlic powder, and minimal salt and pepper.
3. Thread the beef, bell peppers, zucchini, and red onion onto skewers.
4. Grill the skewers, turning occasionally, until the beef is cooked to desired doneness and vegetables are tender, about 8-10 minutes.
5. While the kebabs are grilling, prepare the tzatziki sauce. In a small bowl, combine the Greek yogurt, grated cucumber, minced garlic, lemon juice, and dill. Stir until well mixed.
6. Serve the kebabs with the tzatziki sauce on the side for dipping.

NUTRITION INFORMATION: (APPROXIMATE VALUES PER SERVING): Calories: 310 | Protein: 26g | carbohydrates: 15g | Fats: 16g | Sodium: 200 mg | Potassium: 650 mg | Sugar: 8g | Cholesterol: 60 mg

STIR-FRIED BEEF AND BROCCOLI WITH TAMARI SAUCE

Enjoy this quick and nutritious stir-fried beef with broccoli, flavored with a low-sodium tamari sauce, ideal for a fatty liver diet as it emphasizes lean protein, high fiber, and whole foods.

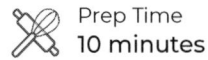

- **Prep Time:** 10 minutes
- **Cooking Time:** 15 minutes
- **Complexity:** Beginner
- **Servings:** 4
- **Ingredients:** 8

EQUIPMENT NEEDED: skillet, mixing bowl, knife, cutting board, measuring cups, measuring spoons

TAGS: High-protein, Whole Foods, Heart-Healthy, Low Glycemic, Low Sodium, High-fiber, Low-fat

INGREDIENT LIST:

- 1 pound lean beef strips (about 450 g)
- 4 cups broccoli florets (about 300 g)
- 1 tablespoon olive oil (15 ml)
- 1/4 cup low-sodium tamari sauce (60 ml), 1 tablespoon freshly grated ginger (15 g)
- 2 cloves garlic, minced (approx. 6 g)
- 1 tablespoon cornstarch (15 ml) mixed with 2 tablespoons water (30 ml)
- 1/2 cup low-sodium beef broth (120 ml)

DIRECTIONS:

1. Heat olive oil in a skillet over medium-high heat.
2. Add garlic and ginger to the skillet, sautéing for about 30 seconds until fragrant.
3. Place beef strips in the skillet and stir-fry until they are browned and nearly cooked through, about 5-7 minutes.
4. Add broccoli and continue to stir-fry for another 5 minutes until the vegetables are tender.
5. In a small bowl, mix the cornstarch and water, then pour into the skillet along with the tamari sauce and beef broth.
6. Stir everything together and cook for another 2-3 minutes until the sauce has thickened and the beef is completely cooked. Serve hot.

NUTRITION INFORMATION: (APPROXIMATE VALUES PER SERVING): Calories: 280 | Protein: 26g | Carbohydrates: 12g | Sodium: 450mg | Fats: 14g | Potassium: 600mg | Sugar: 2g | Cholesterol: 60mg

SPICED CHICKEN SKEWERS WITH YOGURT CUCUMBER DIP

Savor the delightful blend of spiced chicken skewers complemented by a refreshing yogurt cucumber dip tailored for a fatty liver diet with its lean protein and heart-healthy ingredients.

- **Prep Time:** 15 minutes
- **Cooking Time:** 0 minutes
- **Complexity:** Beginner
- **Servings:** 4
- **Ingredients:** 10

EQUIPMENT NEEDED: grill or grill pan, mixing bowl, wooden skewers, knife, cutting board, measuring spoons, measuring cups

TAGS: High-protein, Low Sodium, Low-fat, Heart-Healthy, Whole Foods, High-fiber, Low Glycemic

INGREDIENT LIST:

- 1 pound chicken breast, cut into 1-inch cubes (about 450 g), 1/2 teaspoon ground turmeric (2.5 ml)
- 1 cup plain low-fat Greek yogurt (240 ml), 1 cucumber, finely diced (about 150 g)
- 2 tablespoons fresh lemon juice (30 ml), 1 tablespoon olive oil (15 ml)
- 2 cloves garlic, minced (approx. 6 g)
- 1 teaspoon ground cumin (5 ml)
- 1 teaspoon smoked paprika (5 ml)
- Salt and pepper to taste (minimal)

DIRECTIONS:

1. In a bowl, mix olive oil, lemon juice, garlic, cumin, paprika, turmeric, salt, and pepper. Add chicken cubes to the marinade and toss to coat evenly. Let marinate for at least 30 minutes.
2. Preheat the grill to medium-high heat. Thread the marinated chicken onto wooden skewers.
3. Grill the chicken skewers for 5 minutes on each side or until fully cooked and slightly charred.
4. In another bowl, combine Greek yogurt with diced cucumber, a pinch of salt, and a tablespoon of lemon juice to make the dip.
5. Serve the hot chicken skewers with the yogurt cucumber dip on the side.

NUTRITION INFORMATION: (APPROXIMATE VALUES PER SERVING): Calories: 215 | Protein: 29g | Carbohydrates: 8g | Sodium: 180mg | Fats: 8g | Potassium: 560mg | Sugar: 5g | Cholesterol: 65mg

SPAGHETTI SQUASH AND MEATBALLS WITH TOMATO BASIL SAUCE

Dive into this comforting dish where spaghetti squash replaces traditional pasta, combined with lean meatballs and a fresh tomato basil sauce, perfectly fitting for a fatty liver diet with its focus on high-fiber and low-fat ingredients.

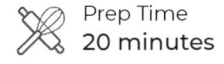

Prep Time: 20 minutes
Cooking Time: 60 minutes
Complexity: Intermediate
Servings: 4
Ingredients: 12

EQUIPMENT NEEDED: oven, skillet, mixing bowl, baking sheet, saucepan, knife, cutting board

TAGS: High-protein, Low Sodium, Low-fat, Heart-Healthy, Whole Foods, High-fiber, Gluten-Free

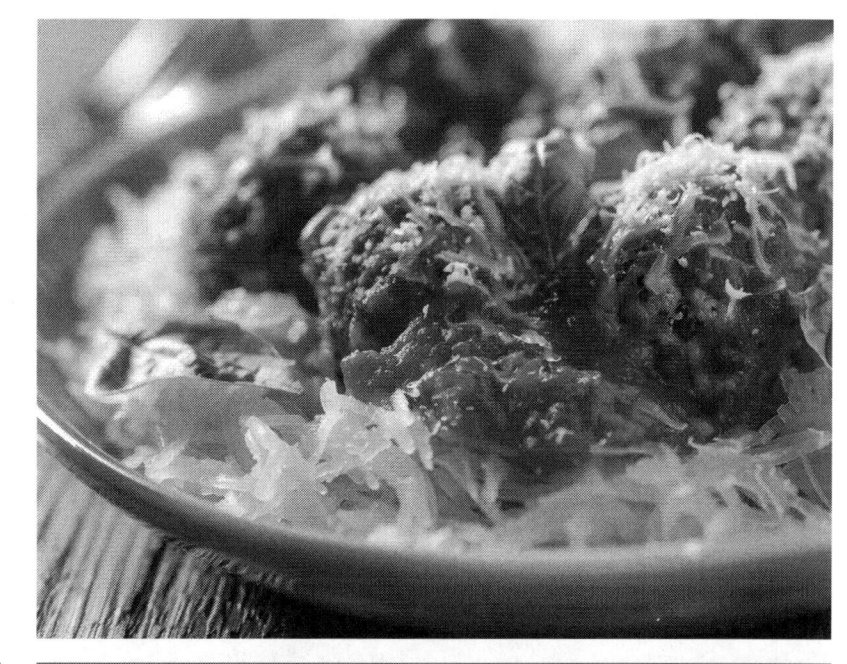

INGREDIENT LIST:

- 1 large spaghetti squash (about 2 pounds, or 900 g)
- 1 pound ground turkey breast (450 g), 1 cup chopped onions (about 150 g), 1/4 cup grated Parmesan cheese (about 30 g)
- 2 cloves garlic, minced (approx. 6 g) 1 egg, beaten, 1/4 cup fresh basil leaves, chopped (about 15 g)
- 1/4 cup fresh parsley, finely chopped (15 g), 2 cups fresh tomatoes, chopped (about 500 g)
- 1 tablespoon olive oil (15 ml)
- Salt and pepper to taste (minimal)
- 1 teaspoon dried oregano (5 ml)

DIRECTIONS:

1. Preheat the oven to 375°F (190°C). Halve the spaghetti squash lengthwise and remove the seeds. Place cut-side down on a baking sheet and bake for 40 minutes until tender.
2. In a mixing bowl, combine ground turkey, half of the chopped onions, garlic, egg, Parmesan, parsley, oregano, salt, and pepper. Form into small meatballs.
3. Heat olive oil in a skillet over medium heat. Add meatballs and cook until browned on all sides and cooked through about 10-15 minutes. Remove and set aside.
4. In the same skillet, add the remaining onions and cook until soft. Add chopped tomatoes and simmer for 20 minutes. Stir in fresh basil and cooked meatballs, simmering for an additional 10 min.
5. Use a fork to scrape the spaghetti squash into strands and divide it among plates. Top with the meatball and tomato basil sauce. Serve hot.

NUTRITION INFORMATION: (APPROXIMATE VALUES PER SERVING): Calories: 330 | Protein: 28g | Carbohydrates: 28g | Sodium: 190mg | Fats: 12g | Potassium: 800mg | Sugar: 12g | Cholesterol: 80mg

CHAPTER 9: FLAVORFUL FISH AND SEAFOOD

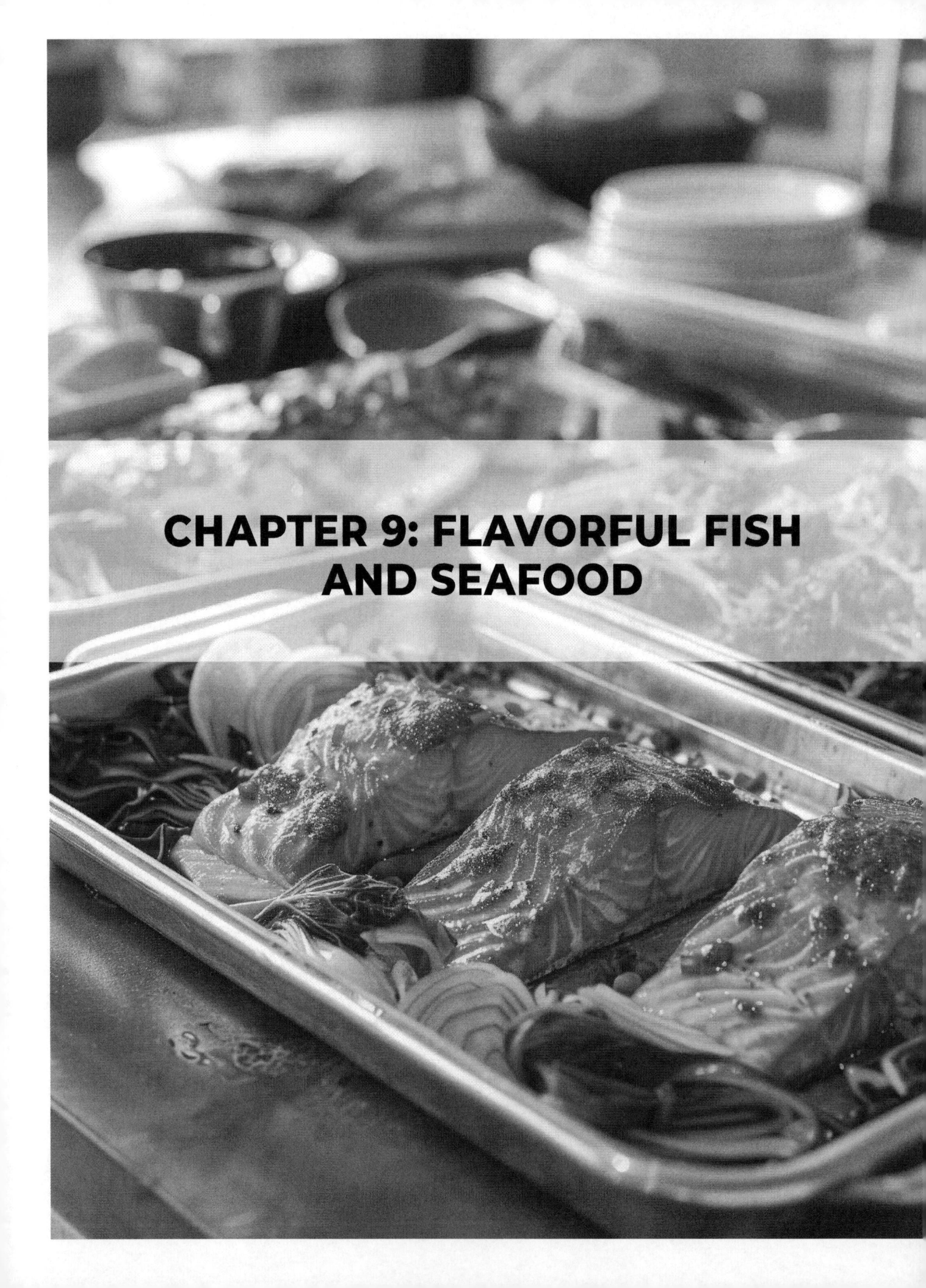

SOY-GINGER GLAZED SALMON WITH BOK CHOY

This dish features omega-rich salmon glazed with a savory soy-ginger sauce and served alongside steamed bok choy, perfectly designed to meet the guidelines of a fatty liver diet with its focus on heart-healthy fats and low glycemic index.

Prep Time: 15 minutes
Cooking Time: 20 minutes
Complexity: Beginner
Servings: 4
Ingredients: 9

EQUIPMENT NEEDED: baking sheet, small saucepan, steamer, mixing bowl, whisk
TAGS: High-protein, Low Sodium, Heart-Healthy, Whole Foods, High-fiber, Low Glycemic, Gluten-Free

INGREDIENT LIST:

- 4 salmon fillets (6 ounces each) (170 g each)
- 2 tablespoons low-sodium soy sauce (30 ml)
- 1 tablespoon grated fresh ginger (15 g), 2 cloves garlic, minced (approx. 6 g)
- 1 tablespoon honey (15 ml)
- 1 tablespoon olive oil (15 ml)
- 4 cups chopped bok choy (about 400 g)
- Salt and pepper to taste (min)
- 1 teaspoon sesame seeds (5 ml) for garnish (optional)

DIRECTIONS:

1. Preheat the oven to 400°F (200°C). Line a baking sheet with parchment paper.
2. In a small saucepan, combine soy sauce, ginger, garlic, and honey. Heat over medium until the mixture just starts to simmer. Remove from heat and stir in olive oil.
3. Place salmon fillets on the prepared baking sheet. Brush each fillet generously with the soy-ginger sauce.
4. Bake the salmon for 12-15 minutes or until cooked through and flakes easily with a fork.
5. While the salmon bakes, steam the chopped bok choy in a steamer for about 5-7 minutes until tender but still crisp.
6. Serve the salmon with steamed bok choy on the side, drizzle any remaining glaze over the top, and sprinkle with sesame seeds if using.

NUTRITION INFORMATION: (APPROXIMATE VALUES PER SERVING): Calories: 295 | Protein: 23g | Carbohydrates: 8g | Sodium: 230mg | Fats: 18g | Potassium: 650mg | Sugar: 5g | Cholesterol: 55mg

PARCHMENT-BAKED HALIBUT WITH ASPARAGUS

This heart-healthy dish features parchment-baked halibut paired with asparagus, seasoned with herbs and lemon, delivering a low-fat, high-protein meal perfect for supporting liver health and overall wellness.

Prep Time: 10 minutes
Cooking Time: 20 minutes
Complexity: Beginner
Servings: 4
Ingredients: 6

EQUIPMENT NEEDED: oven, parchment paper, baking sheet, knife, cutting board
TAGS: High-protein, Low Sodium, Heart-Healthy, Whole Foods, High-fiber, Low-fat, Gluten-Free

INGREDIENT LIST:

- 4 halibut fillets (6 ounces each) (170 g each)
- 1 pound asparagus, trimmed (450 g)
- 2 tablespoons olive oil (30 ml)
- 1 lemon, sliced (approx. 120 g)
- Salt and pepper to taste (minimal)
- 4 sprigs fresh dill (or 1 teaspoon dried dill) (5 ml)

DIRECTIONS:

1. Preheat the oven to 400°F (200°C). Cut four pieces of parchment paper large enough to wrap each fillet and a portion of asparagus.
2. Place a halibut fillet and a quarter of the asparagus in the center of each piece of parchment. Drizzle with olive oil and season with salt and pepper. Top each with lemon slices and a sprig of dill.
3. Fold the parchment paper over the ingredients, twisting the ends to seal into a packet.
4. Place the packets on a baking sheet and bake for 15-20 minutes, until the halibut is cooked through and the asparagus is tender.
5. Carefully open the packets (watch for steam) and serve immediately.

NUTRITION INFORMATION: (APPROXIMATE VALUES PER SERVING): Calories: 280 | Protein: 31g | Carbohydrates: 6g | Sodium: 70mg | Fats: 15g | Potassium: 800mg | Sugar: 2g | Cholesterol: 55mg

HORSERADISH ENCRUSTED SALMON WITH BEETROOT SALAD

This vibrant dish features omega-3-rich salmon encrusted with a tangy horseradish topping, paired with a refreshing beetroot salad, perfectly tailored to support liver health and overall wellness.

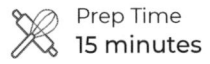

Prep Time: 15 minutes
Cooking Time: 20 minutes
Complexity: Beginner
Servings: 4
Ingredients: 9

EQUIPMENT NEEDED: oven, baking sheet, mixing bowl, salad bowl, knife, cutting board

TAGS: High-protein, Low Sodium, Heart-Healthy, Whole Foods, High-fiber, Low Glycemic, Gluten-Free

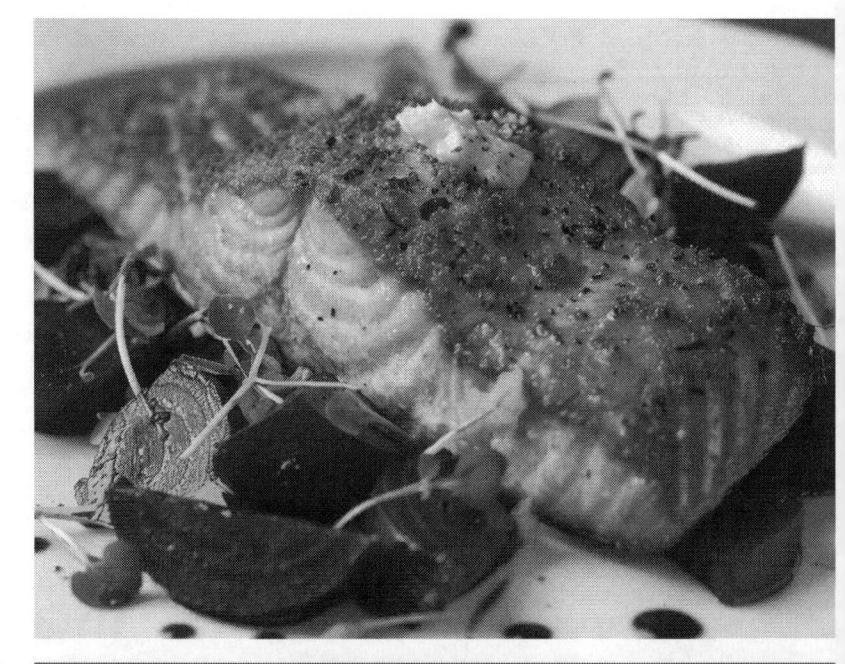

INGREDIENT LIST:

- 4 salmon fillets (6 ounces each) (170 g each)
- 2 tablespoons prepared horseradish (30 ml)
- 1 tablespoon Dijon mustard (15 ml)
- 1 tablespoon olive oil (15 ml)
- 2 medium beetroots, cooked and sliced (about 150 g each)
- 2 cups arugula (about 60 g)
- 1 tablespoon balsamic vinegar (15 ml)
- 1 tablespoon lemon juice (15 ml)
- Salt and pepper to taste (minimal)

DIRECTIONS:

1. Preheat the oven to 400°F (200°C). Line a baking sheet with parchment paper.
2. In a small bowl, mix the horseradish, Dijon mustard, and a pinch of salt and pepper.
3. Place the salmon fillets on the prepared baking sheet. Spread the horseradish mixture evenly over the top of each fillet.
4. Bake in the oven for 15-18 minutes or until the salmon is cooked through and the topping is slightly golden.
5. While the salmon cooks, prepare the beetroot salad. In a salad bowl, toss the sliced beetroots with arugula, balsamic vinegar, olive oil, and lemon juice.
6. Serve the cooked salmon with the beetroot salad on the side.

NUTRITION INFORMATION: (APPROXIMATE VALUES PER SERVING): Calories: 280 | Protein: 24g | Carbohydrates: 10g | Sodium: 180mg | Fats: 16g | Potassium: 800mg | Sugar: 7g | Cholesterol: 55mg

LEMON-PEPPER COD WITH BROCCOLI PUREE

Enjoy this delicate and nutritious Lemon-Pepper Cod paired with a creamy broccoli puree. This dish is designed to fit a fatty liver diet by offering high-protein, high-fiber, and low-fat content with minimal sodium, ensuring a healthy yet flavorful meal.

- Prep Time: 10 minutes
- Cooking Time: 20 minutes
- Complexity: Beginner
- Servings: 4
- Ingredients: 7

EQUIPMENT NEEDED: baking sheet, steamer, blender, oven, knife, cutting board
TAGS: High-protein, Low Sodium, Heart-Healthy, Whole Foods, High-fiber, Low-fat, Gluten-Free, Low Glycemic

INGREDIENT LIST:

- 4 cod fillets (6 ounces each) (170 g each)
- 2 tablespoons olive oil (30 ml)
- 1 lemon, zest and juice (approx. 120 g)
- 1 teaspoon black pepper (5 ml)
- 4 cups broccoli florets (about 360 g)
- Salt to taste (minimal)
- 1 clove garlic, minced (approx. 3 g)

DIRECTIONS:

1. Preheat the oven to 375°F (190°C). Line a baking sheet with parchment paper. Place the cod fillets on the prepared baking sheet. Drizzle each with olive oil and lemon juice, then season with lemon zest, black pepper, and a pinch of salt.
2. Bake the cod in the oven for 12-15 minutes or until the fish flakes easily with a fork. While the cod is baking, steam the broccoli florets for about 7-10 minutes until very tender.
3. Transfer the steamed broccoli to a blender, add the minced garlic, and blend until smooth. If needed, add a little water to achieve a creamy consistency.
4. Serve the baked cod over a bed of broccoli puree.

NUTRITION INFORMATION: (APPROXIMATE VALUES PER SERVING): Calories: 220 | Protein: 25g | Carbohydrates: 8g | Sodium: 70mg | Fats: 10g | Potassium: 650mg | Sugar: 2g | Cholesterol: 60mg

MAPLE-GLAZED ARCTIC CHAR WITH BRAISED LEEKS

Delight in the sweet and savory blend of maple-glazed Arctic char, accompanied by gently braised leeks. This dish combines the heart-healthy benefits of omega-rich fish with the gentle sweetness of maple, suitable for a fatty liver diet.

- Prep Time: 15 minutes
- Cooking Time: 25 minutes
- Complexity: Intermediate
- Servings: 4
- Ingredients: 7

EQUIPMENT NEEDED: oven, skillet, baking sheet, knife, cutting board
TAGS: High-protein, Low Sodium, Heart-Healthy, Whole Foods, High-fiber, Low-fat, Gluten-Free

INGREDIENT LIST:

- 4 Arctic char fillets (6 ounces each) (170 g each)
- 2 tablespoons pure maple syrup (30 ml)
- 1 tablespoon Dijon mustard (15 ml)
- 2 large leeks, white and light green parts only, sliced and rinsed (about 200 g)
- 2 tablespoons olive oil (30 ml)
- Salt and pepper to taste (minimal)
- 1/4 cup low-sodium vegetable broth (60 ml)

DIRECTIONS:

1. Preheat the oven to 375°F (190°C). Line a baking sheet with parchment paper.
2. In a small bowl, mix the maple syrup and Dijon mustard. Brush the mixture over the Arctic char fillets.
3. Place the glazed fillets on the prepared baking sheet. Season with a pinch of salt and pepper.
4. Bake in the oven for 15-20 minutes or until the fish is opaque and flakes easily with a fork.
5. While the fish is baking, heat olive oil in a skillet over medium heat. Add the sliced leeks and sauté until they begin to soften, about 5 minutes.
6. Add the vegetable broth to the skillet, reduce the heat to low, cover, and let the leeks braise until they are tender, about 10-15 minutes.
7. Serve the maple-glazed Arctic char with a side of braised leeks.

NUTRITION INFORMATION: (APPROXIMATE VALUES PER SERVING): Calories: 330 | Protein: 25g | Carbohydrates: 10g | Sodium: 180mg | Fats: 20g | Potassium: 650mg | Sugar: 7g | Cholesterol: 55mg

SPICED MONKFISH WITH LENTIL DAL

Enjoy a fusion of flavors with this spiced monkfish paired with a creamy lentil dal, offering a nutrient-rich meal that supports liver health with its high protein and fiber content.

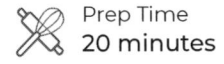

Prep Time: 20 minutes
Cooking Time: 40 minutes
Complexity: Intermediate
Servings: 4
Ingredients: 12

EQUIPMENT NEEDED: sauté pan, pot, knife, cutting board, measuring spoons, measuring cups

TAGS: High-protein, High-fiber, Low Sodium, Heart-Healthy, Whole Foods, Low Glycemic, Gluten-Free

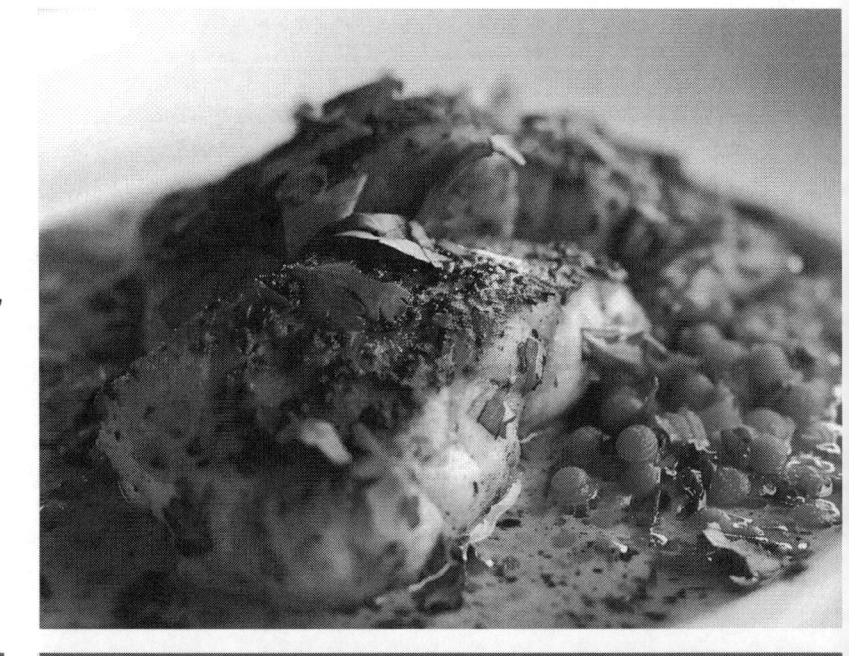

INGREDIENT LIST:

- 4 monkfish fillets (6 ounces each) (170 g each)
- 1 tablespoon olive oil (15 ml)
- 1 teaspoon ground turmeric (5 ml)
- 1 teaspoon ground cumin (5 ml)
- 1 teaspoon ground coriander (5 ml)
- 1 cup red lentils, rinsed (190 g)
- 4 cups low-sodium vegetable broth (960 ml)
- 1 large onion, finely chopped (about 150 g)
- 2 cloves garlic, minced (approx. 6 g)
- 1 tablespoon grated ginger (15 g)
- 1 teaspoon garam masala (5 ml)
- Salt and pepper to taste (minimal)

DIRECTIONS:

1. Heat olive oil in a sauté pan over medium heat. Add turmeric, cumin, and coriander; stir for 30 seconds to release the flavors.
2. Add monkfish fillets to the pan, season with salt and pepper, and cook for 4-5 minutes on each side until the fish is cooked through and lightly browned. Remove and set aside.
3. In the same pan, add more oil if needed, and sauté onion, garlic, and ginger until onion is translucent, about 5 minutes.
4. Add lentils and vegetable broth to the pan. Bring to a boil, then reduce heat and simmer for 20-25 minutes, or until lentils are soft and the mixture has thickened.
5. Stir in garam masala and season with salt and pepper to taste.
6. Serve the spiced monkfish over a bed of creamy lentil dal.

NUTRITION INFORMATION: (APPROXIMATE VALUES PER SERVING): Calories: 370 | Protein: 36g | Carbohydrates: 38g | Sodium: 200mg | Fats: 7g | Potassium: 950mg | Sugar: 4g | Cholesterol: 45mg

STEAMED MUSSELS WITH GARLIC AND HERBS

Savor the natural sweetness and delicate texture of mussels steamed with aromatic garlic and herbs. This dish is ideal for a fatty liver diet, offering high protein with minimal fats and controlled sodium levels.

- **Prep Time:** 10 minutes
- **Cooking Time:** 10 minutes
- **Complexity:** Beginner
- **Servings:** 4
- **Ingredients:** 7

EQUIPMENT NEEDED: large pot, knife, cutting board, measuring spoons
TAGS: High-protein, Low Sodium, Heart-Healthy, Whole Foods, Low Glycemic, Gluten-Free, Low-fat

INGREDIENT LIST:

- 2 pounds fresh mussels, cleaned and debearded (about 900 g)
- 2 tablespoons olive oil (30 ml)
- 4 cloves garlic, minced (approx. 12 g)
- 1/2 cup low-sodium vegetable broth (120 ml)
- 1/4 cup chopped fresh parsley (15 g)
- 1 lemon, juiced (approx. 45 ml)
- Fresh ground black pepper to taste

DIRECTIONS:

1. In a large pot, heat the olive oil over medium heat. Add the minced garlic and sauté for about 1 minute until fragrant, being careful not to burn it.
2. Pour in the vegetable broth and bring to a simmer.
3. Add the mussels to the pot, cover, and let steam for about 5-7 minutes until all mussels have opened. Discard any mussels that do not open.
4. Once cooked, stir in the fresh lemon juice and chopped parsley, and season with fresh ground black pepper.
5. Serve the mussels hot, ensuring to spoon some of the broth over the mussels in each bowl.

NUTRITION INFORMATION: (APPROXIMATE VALUES PER SERVING): Calories: 195 | Protein: 18g | Carbohydrates: 6g | Sodium: 290mg | Fats: 10g | Potassium: 380mg | Sugar: 0g | Cholesterol: 48mg

LEMON AND DILL POACHED SALMON

Experience the freshness of lemon and dill in this delicately poached salmon dish, perfectly suited for a fatty liver diet with its focus on heart-healthy fats and lean protein.

- **Prep Time:** 10 minutes
- **Cooking Time:** 15 minutes
- **Complexity:** Beginner
- **Servings:** 4
- **Ingredients:** 6

EQUIPMENT NEEDED: pot, knife, cutting board, measuring spoons
TAGS: High-protein, Low Sodium, Heart-Healthy, Whole Foods, Low Glycemic, Low-fat, Gluten-Free, Low-calorie

INGREDIENT LIST:

- 4 salmon fillets (6 ounces each) (170 g each)
- 4 cups water (960 ml)
- 2 lemons, one juiced and one sliced (approx. 120 g each)
- 4 sprigs fresh dill (or 1 tablespoon dried dill) (15 ml)
- 1 teaspoon black peppercorns (5 ml)
- Salt to taste (minimal)

DIRECTIONS:

1. Fill a large pot with the water and bring to a simmer over medium heat. Add the lemon juice, half of the lemon slices, dill sprigs, peppercorns, and a pinch of salt.
2. Gently place the salmon fillets in the simmering water, ensuring they are fully submerged. Adjust the heat to maintain a gentle simmer and poach the salmon for about 10-12 minutes or until cooked through and opaque.
3. Carefully remove the salmon from the water with a slotted spoon and place it on serving plates.
4. Garnish each fillet with the remaining lemon slices and a sprig of fresh dill.
5. Serve immediately while warm.

NUTRITION INFORMATION: (APPROXIMATE VALUES PER SERVING): Calories: 200 | Protein: 23g | Carbohydrates: 2g | Sodium: 50mg | Fats: 12g | Potassium: 500mg | Sugar: 1g | Cholesterol: 60mg

GRILLED TUNA WITH A CITRUS TOMATO SALSA

This grilled tuna steak served with a vibrant citrus tomato salsa, is a perfect example of a heart-healthy, high-protein dish designed for a fatty liver diet, focusing on lean protein and fresh, nutrient-rich ingredients.

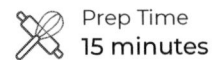

Prep Time: 15 minutes
Cooking Time: 10 minutes
Complexity: Beginner
Servings: 4
Ingredients: 9

EQUIPMENT NEEDED: grill or grill pan, mixing bowl, knife, cutting board, measuring spoons, measuring cups
TAGS: High-protein, Low Sodium, Heart-Healthy, Whole Foods, Low Glycemic, Gluten-Free, Low-fat

INGREDIENT LIST:

- 4 tuna steaks (6 ounces each) (170 g each), 2 large tomatoes, diced (about 200 g each)
- 2 tablespoons olive oil (30 ml)
- Salt and pepper to taste (min)
- 1 orange, segmented and chopped (approx. 140 g)
- 1 lime, juiced (approx. 30 ml)
- 1 small red onion, finely chopped (about 70 g), 1/4 cup chopped fresh cilantro (15 g)
- 1 jalapeño, seeded and finely chopped (optional, adjust to taste) (about 15 g)

DIRECTIONS:

1. Preheat the grill or grill pan to medium-high heat.
2. Brush the tuna steaks lightly with one tablespoon of olive oil and season with salt and pepper.
3. Grill the tuna steaks for about 2-3 minutes on each side or until desired doneness is reached.
4. In a mixing bowl, combine the diced tomatoes, orange segments, lime juice, red onion, cilantro, jalapeño (if using), and the remaining tablespoon of olive oil. Season with salt and pepper to taste and mix well to combine.
5. Serve the grilled tuna steaks topped with the citrus tomato salsa.

NUTRITION INFORMATION: (APPROXIMATE VALUES PER SERVING): Calories: 290 | Protein: 27g | Carbohydrates: 9g | Sodium: 180mg | Fats: 16g | Potassium: 500mg | Sugar: 6g | Cholesterol: 45mg

MISO GLAZED BLACK COD WITH STIR-FRIED GREENS

This recipe features succulent black cod with a savory miso glaze, complemented by a side of lightly stir-fried greens, creating a dish rich in omega-3 fatty acids and dietary fiber, perfect for those following a fatty liver diet.

Prep Time: 20 minutes
Cooking Time: 15 minutes
Complexity: Intermediate
Servings: 4
Ingredients: 9

EQUIPMENT NEEDED: oven, baking sheet, skillet, mixing bowl, brush
TAGS: High-protein, Low Sodium, Heart-Healthy, Whole Foods, Low Glycemic, Gluten-Free, High-fiber

INGREDIENT LIST:

- 4 black cod fillets (6 ounces each) (170 g each), 2 tablespoons white miso paste (30 ml)
- 1 tablespoon mirin (15 ml)
- 1 tablespoon sake (15 ml)
- 1 tablespoon soy sauce, low sodium (15 ml)
- 1 teaspoon sesame oil (5 ml)
- 4 cups mixed greens (spinach, kale, Swiss chard) (about 360 g)
- 2 cloves garlic, minced (approx. 6 g)
- 1 tablespoon ginger, freshly grated (15 g)

DIRECTIONS:

1. Preheat the oven to 400°F (200°C). Line a baking sheet with parchment paper. In a small bowl, mix together the miso paste, mirin, sake, and soy sauce to create the glaze.
2. Place the cod fillets on the prepared baking sheet. Brush each fillet generously with the miso glaze.
3. Bake in the preheated oven for about 12-15 minutes or until the fish flakes easily with a fork.
4. While the fish is baking, heat the sesame oil in a skillet over medium heat. Add the minced garlic and grated ginger, sautéing for about 1 minute until fragrant.
5. Add the mixed greens to the skillet, stirring frequently, until the greens are just wilted, about 3-4 minutes. Serve the miso-glazed black cod with the stir-fried greens on the side.

NUTRITION INFORMATION: (APPROXIMATE VALUES PER SERVING): Calories: 280 | Protein: 28g | Carbohydrates: 10g | Sodium: 340mg | Fats: 12g | Potassium: 800mg | Sugar: 2g | Cholesterol: 55mg

CHAPTER 10: DESSERTS

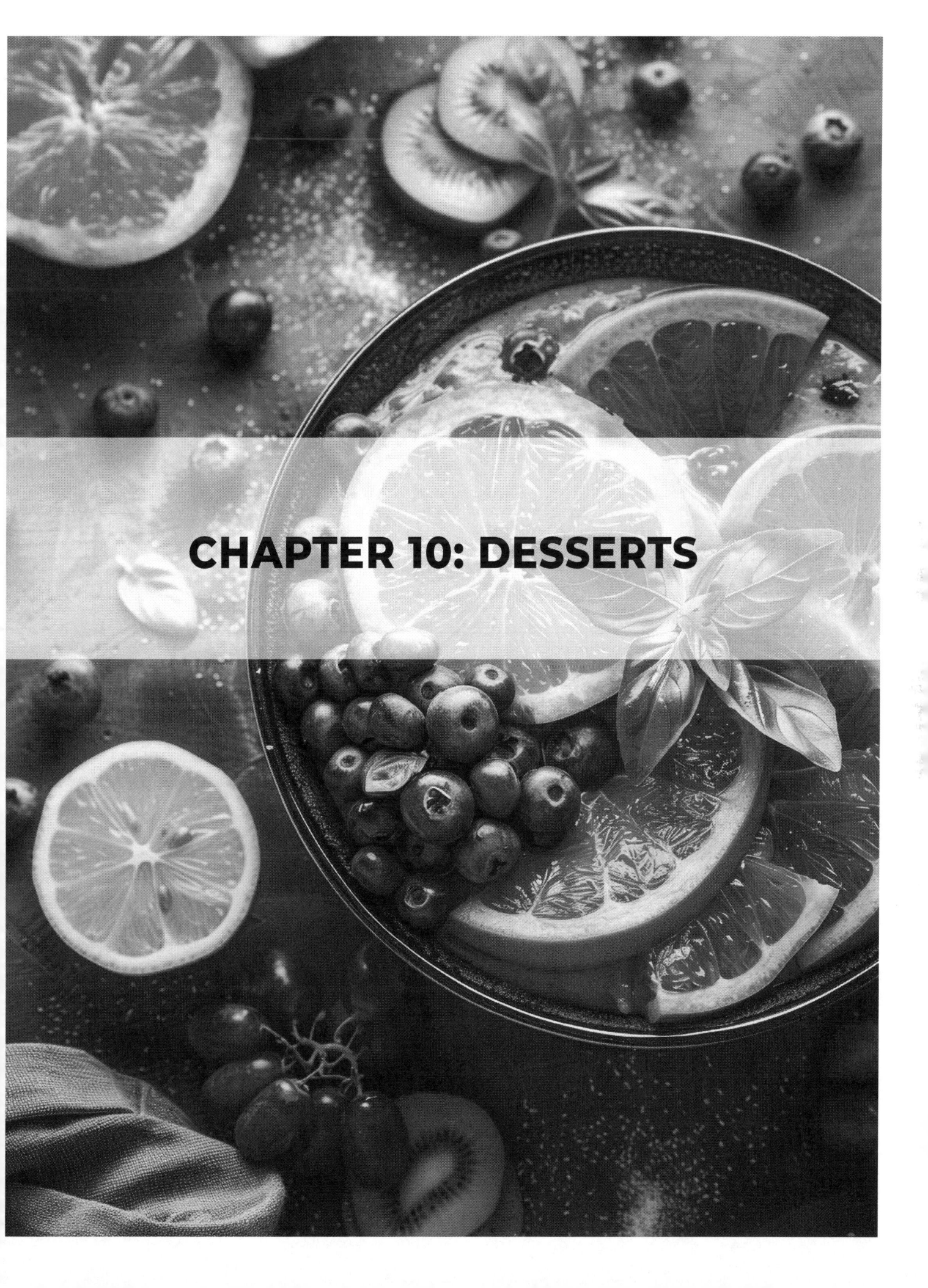

PUMPKIN SPICE ENERGY BALLS

These no-bake Pumpkin Spice Energy Balls are a delicious and nutritious snack, perfect for meeting the dietary needs of those with a fatty liver. Packed with fiber, healthy fats, and a hint of sweetness, they are ideal for an energy boost without added sugars.

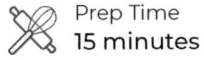

Prep Time: 15 minutes
Cooking Time: 0 minutes
Complexity: Beginner
Servings: 12
Ingredients: 7

EQUIPMENT NEEDED: food processor, measuring cups, measuring spoons, mixing bowl
TAGS: High-fiber, Low Sodium, Heart-Healthy, Whole Foods, Low Glycemic, Gluten-Free, Vegetarian, Dairy-Free, Low-fat

INGREDIENT LIST:

- 1 cup rolled oats (gluten-free if necessary) (90 g)
- 1/2 cup pumpkin puree (about 120 g)
- 1/4 cup ground flax seeds (30 g)
- 1/4 cup almond butter (60 ml)
- 2 tablespoons honey (substitute with agave syrup for vegan option) (30 ml)
- 1 teaspoon pumpkin pie spice (5 ml)
- 1/4 cup chopped pecans or walnuts (optional for extra crunch) (30 g)

DIRECTIONS:

1. In a food processor, combine the rolled oats, pumpkin puree, ground flax seeds, almond butter, honey (or agave), and pumpkin pie spice. Pulse until the mixture is well combined and begins to stick together.
2. Transfer the mixture to a mixing bowl. If using, stir in the chopped nuts.
3. Using your hands, roll the mixture into small balls about 1 inch in diameter.
4. Place the energy balls on a plate or baking sheet lined with parchment paper.
5. Refrigerate for at least 30 minutes to set before serving. Store in an airtight container in the refrigerator.

NUTRITION INFORMATION: (APPROXIMATE VALUES PER SERVING): Calories: 110 | Protein: 3g | Carbohydrates: 12g | Sodium: 5mg | Fats: 6g | Potassium: 115mg | Sugar: 4g | Cholesterol: 0mg

PINEAPPLE CARPACCIO WITH FRESH BASIL

This refreshing Pineapple Carpaccio with Fresh Basil is a simple yet elegant dessert that aligns with the fatty liver diet, emphasizing whole, nutrient-dense ingredients with natural sweetness and rich in vitamins.

Prep Time: 15 minutes
Cooking Time: 0 minutes
Complexity: Beginner
Servings: 4
Ingredients: 4

EQUIPMENT NEEDED: sharp knife, cutting board, mixing bowl, serving plates
TAGS: Whole Foods, Vegan, Low Glycemic, Heart-Healthy, Gluten-Free, Dairy-Free, Low Sodium, Low-fat, Low-calorie, Vitamin C rich

INGREDIENT LIST:

- 1 large ripe pineapple, peeled and cored
- 1/4 cup fresh basil leaves, thinly sliced (about 15 g)
- Juice of 1 lime (about 2 tablespoons, 30 ml)
- 1 tablespoon honey (optional, skip for sugar-free needs) (15 ml)

DIRECTIONS:

1. Using a sharp knife, slice the pineapple into very thin rounds. Arrange the slices in a single layer on serving plates.
2. In a small bowl, mix the lime juice and honey (if using) until well combined.
3. Drizzle the lime and honey mixture over the pineapple slices.
4. Sprinkle the thinly sliced basil leaves over the top of the pineapple slices just before serving.

NUTRITION INFORMATION: (APPROXIMATE VALUES PER SERVING): Calories: 100 | Protein: 1g | Carbohydrates: 25g | Sodium: 2mg | Fats: 0g | Potassium: 215mg | Sugar: 19g | Cholesterol: 0mg

AVOCADO COCOA MOUSSE

This Avocado Cocoa Mousse is a creamy and delicious dessert that fits perfectly into a fatty liver diet, providing a rich source of healthy fats from avocado and a natural sweetness without added sugars.

- **Prep Time:** 10 minutes
- **Cooking Time:** 0 minutes
- **Complexity:** Beginner
- **Servings:** 4
- **Ingredients:** 5

EQUIPMENT NEEDED: blender, measuring spoons, measuring cups, mixing bowl

TAGS: Vegan, Gluten-Free, Dairy-Free, Low Glycemic, Heart-Healthy, Whole Foods, High-fiber, Low Sodium, Low-fat

INGREDIENT LIST:

- 2 ripe avocados, peeled and pitted (about 200 g each)
- 1/4 cup unsweetened cocoa powder (about 30 g)
- 2 tablespoons pure maple syrup (or agave syrup for a lower glycemic index) (30 ml)
- 1 teaspoon pure vanilla extract (5 ml)
- A pinch of salt

DIRECTIONS:

1. Place the avocados, cocoa powder, maple syrup, vanilla extract, and a pinch of salt in a blender.
2. Blend on high until the mixture is completely smooth. If the mixture is too thick, add a little water, one tablespoon at a time, to reach the desired consistency.
3. Taste and adjust the sweetness by adding a little more maple syrup if needed.
4. Transfer the mousse to a mixing bowl and refrigerate for at least 30 minutes to thicken slightly and chill.
5. Serve the mousse chilled, optionally garnished with fresh fruit or a sprinkle of cocoa powder.

NUTRITION INFORMATION: (APPROXIMATE VALUES PER SERVING): Calories: 230 | Protein: 3g | Carbohydrates: 20g | Sodium: 10mg | Fats: 16g | Potassium: 487mg | Sugar: 8g | Cholesterol: 0mg

BAKED GRAPEFRUIT WITH CINNAMON

This warm and slightly caramelized Baked Grapefruit with Cinnamon offers a delightful and healthy dessert option. Rich in Vitamin C and low in calories, this simple dish satisfies the sweet tooth while adhering to a fatty liver diet, using natural fruit sugars and beneficial spices.

- **Prep Time:** 5 minutes
- **Cooking Time:** 15 minutes
- **Complexity:** Beginner
- **Servings:** 2
- **Ingredients:** 3

EQUIPMENT NEEDED: oven, baking sheet, knife, cutting board

TAGS: Whole Foods, Vegan, Gluten-Free, Dairy-Free, Low Glycemic, Heart-Healthy, Low Sodium, Low-fat, Low-calorie, Vitamin C rich

INGREDIENT LIST:

- 1 large grapefruit, halved (about 250 g per half)
- 1 teaspoon ground cinnamon (5 ml)
- 1 tablespoon honey (optional; omit for sugar-free version) (15 ml)

DIRECTIONS:

1. Preheat the oven to 375°F (190°C).
2. Place the grapefruit halves on a baking sheet, cut-side up.
3. Sprinkle each half evenly with ground cinnamon, and drizzle with honey if using.
4. Bake in the preheated oven for 15 minutes or until the tops are slightly caramelized and the grapefruit is warm.
5. Allow to cool slightly before serving.

NUTRITION INFORMATION: (APPROXIMATE VALUES PER SERVING): Calories: 52 | Protein: 1g | Carbohydrates: 13g | Sodium: 0mg | Fats: 0g | Potassium: 166mg | Sugar: 11g (natural sugars from grapefruit) | Cholesterol: 0mg

PEAR AND GINGER COMPOTE

This Pear and Ginger Compote is a warm, soothing dessert that aligns with the fatty liver diet by using natural, fiber-rich ingredients to provide a low-calorie sweet treat without added sugars.

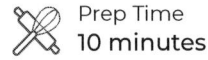

- **Prep Time:** 10 minutes
- **Cooking Time:** 20 minutes
- **Complexity:** Beginner
- **Servings:** 4
- **Ingredients:** 5

EQUIPMENT NEEDED: saucepan, knife, cutting board, measuring spoons

TAGS: Whole Foods, Vegan, Gluten-Free, Dairy-Free, Low Glycemic, Heart-Healthy, Low Sodium, High-fiber, Low-fat, Low-calorie, Vitamin C rich

INGREDIENT LIST:

- 4 ripe pears, peeled, cored, and chopped (about 150 g each)
- 2 tablespoons freshly grated ginger (30 ml)
- 1 cinnamon stick (or 1 teaspoon ground cinnamon) (5 ml)
- Juice of 1 lemon (about 2 tablespoons, 30 ml)
- 1 cup water (240 ml)

DIRECTIONS:

1. In a saucepan over medium heat, combine the chopped pears, grated ginger, cinnamon stick, lemon juice, and water.
2. Bring the mixture to a simmer and cook for about 20 minutes, or until the pears are very soft and the mixture has thickened slightly.
3. Remove the cinnamon stick (if used) and mash the mixture slightly with a fork to create a chunky compote.
4. Serve warm, or let cool and store in the refrigerator to serve chilled.

NUTRITION INFORMATION: (APPROXIMATE VALUES PER SERVING): Calories: 120 | Protein: 1g | Carbohydrates: 31g | Sodium: 2mg | Fats: 0g | Potassium: 200mg | Sugar: 20g (natural sugars from pears) | Cholesterol: 0mg

ROASTED CINNAMON HAZELNUTS

These Roasted Cinnamon Hazelnuts are a delightful, crunchy snack that aligns with a fatty liver diet, offering a heart-healthy, high-protein treat with minimal added sugars. This recipe enhances the natural flavors of hazelnuts with a touch of cinnamon, making it an ideal dessert or snack.

- **Prep Time:** 5 minutes
- **Cooking Time:** 10 minutes
- **Complexity:** Beginner
- **Servings:** 4
- **Ingredients:** 3

EQUIPMENT NEEDED: baking sheet, oven, mixing bowl, spoon

TAGS: Whole Foods, Vegan, Gluten-Free, Dairy-Free, Low Glycemic, Heart-Healthy, High-fiber, Low Sodium, Low-fat, Low-calorie

INGREDIENT LIST:

- 1 cup hazelnuts (about 135 g)
- 1 teaspoon ground cinnamon (5 ml)
- 1 tablespoon maple syrup (optional, for a touch of sweetness) (15 ml)

DIRECTIONS:

1. Preheat the oven to 350°F (175°C).
2. In a mixing bowl, combine the hazelnuts, cinnamon, and maple syrup if using. Stir until the hazelnuts are evenly coated.
3. Spread the hazelnuts in a single layer on a baking sheet.
4. Roast in the preheated oven for about 10 minutes or until the hazelnuts are golden and fragrant. Stir halfway through to ensure even roasting.
5. Remove from the oven and let cool. The hazelnuts will become crunchier as they cool.
6. Serve as a snack or use as a topping for salads or desserts.

NUTRITION INFORMATION: (APPROXIMATE VALUES PER SERVING): Calories: 178 | Protein: 4g | Carbohydrates: 6g | Sodium: 0mg | Fats: 17g | Potassium: 200mg | Sugar: 1g | Cholesterol: 0mg

BLUEBERRY AND LEMON CHIA FRESCA

This refreshing Blueberry and Lemon Chia Fresca is a hydrating drink packed with antioxidants and fiber, perfect for supporting liver health and digestion. It combines the natural sweetness of blueberries with the zest of lemon, enhanced with the nutritional powerhouse of chia seeds.

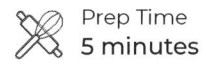

Prep Time: 5 minutes
Cooking Time: 0 minutes
Complexity: Beginner
Servings: 2
Ingredients: 5

EQUIPMENT NEEDED: mixing bowl, spoon, glasses

TAGS: Whole Foods, Vegan, Gluten-Free, Dairy-Free, Low Glycemic, Heart-Healthy, High-fiber, Low Sodium, Low-fat, Low-calorie, Vitamin C rich

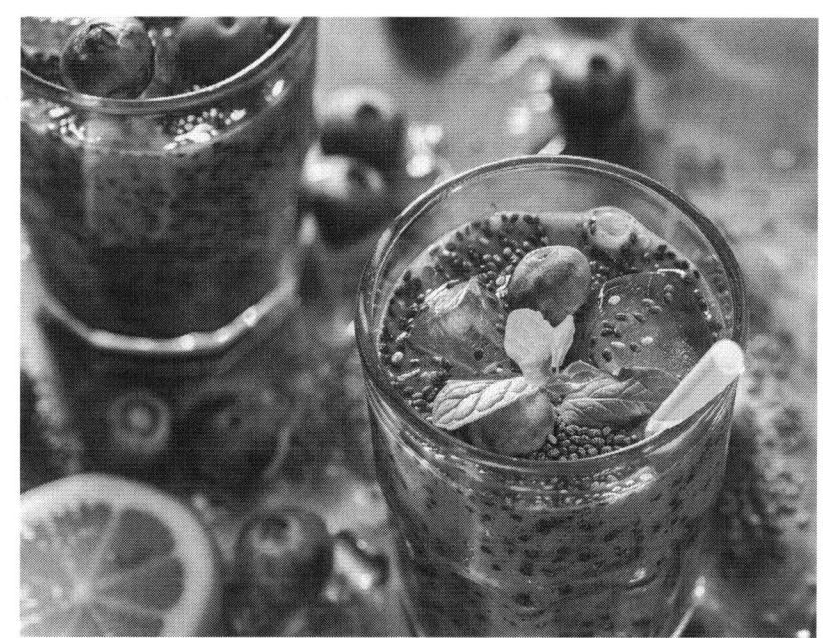

INGREDIENT LIST:

- 4 monkfish fillets (6 ounces each) (170 g each)
- 1 tablespoon olive oil (15 ml)
- 1 teaspoon ground turmeric (5 ml)
- 1 teaspoon ground cumin (5 ml)
- 1 teaspoon ground coriander (5 ml)
- 1 cup red lentils, rinsed (190 g)
- 4 cups low-sodium vegetable broth (960 ml)
- 1 large onion, finely chopped (about 150 g)
- 2 cloves garlic, minced (approx. 6 g)
- 1 tablespoon grated ginger (15 g)
- 1 teaspoon garam masala (5 ml)
- Salt and pepper to taste (minimal)

DIRECTIONS:

1. Heat olive oil in a sauté pan over medium heat. Add turmeric, cumin, and coriander; stir for 30 seconds to release the flavors.
2. Add monkfish fillets to the pan, season with salt and pepper, and cook for 4-5 minutes on each side until the fish is cooked through and lightly browned. Remove and set aside.
3. In the same pan, add more oil if needed, and sauté onion, garlic, and ginger until onion is translucent, about 5 minutes.
4. Add lentils and vegetable broth to the pan. Bring to a boil, then reduce heat and simmer for 20-25 minutes, or until lentils are soft and the mixture has thickened.
5. Stir in garam masala and season with salt and pepper to taste.
6. Serve the spiced monkfish over a bed of creamy lentil dal.

NUTRITION INFORMATION: (APPROXIMATE VALUES PER SERVING): Calories: 60 | Protein: 2g | Carbohydrates: 10g | Sodium: 5mg | Fats: 2g | Potassium: 80mg | Sugar: 4g (natural sugars from blueberries) | Cholesterol: 0mg

RASPBERRY COCONUT CHIA PUDDING

This Raspberry Coconut Chia Pudding is a vibrant and nutritious dessert that perfectly complements a fatty liver diet. It combines the richness of coconut with the tartness of raspberries and the nutritional benefits of chia seeds to create a satisfying dessert that's high in fiber and essential nutrients.

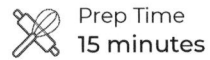

- **Prep Time:** 15 minutes
- **Cooking Time:** 0 minutes
- **Complexity:** Beginner
- **Servings:** 4
- **Ingredients:** 5

EQUIPMENT NEEDED: mixing bowl, whisk, serving glasses

TAGS: Whole Foods, Vegan, Gluten-Free, Dairy-Free, Low Glycemic, Heart-Healthy, High-fiber, Low Sodium, Low-fat, Low-calorie, Vitamin C rich

INGREDIENT LIST:

- 1/4 cup chia seeds (about 40 g)
- 1 cup unsweetened coconut milk (240 ml)
- 1 cup fresh raspberries (about 123 g)
- 1 tablespoon maple syrup (optional, for added sweetness) (15 ml)
- 1/2 teaspoon vanilla extract (2.5 ml)

DIRECTIONS:

1. In a mixing bowl, combine the chia seeds and coconut milk. Whisk thoroughly to prevent clumping.
2. Stir in the vanilla extract and maple syrup if using.
3. Gently fold in the fresh raspberries, reserving a few for topping.
4. Divide the mixture evenly among four serving glasses.
5. Refrigerate for at least 4 hours or overnight, allowing the chia seeds to absorb the liquid and thicken into a pudding consistency.
6. Before serving, top each pudding with the reserved raspberries for added freshness and visual appeal.

NUTRITION INFORMATION: (APPROXIMATE VALUES PER SERVING): Calories: 140 | Protein: 3g | Carbohydrates: 12g | Sodium: 15mg | Fats: 9g | Potassium: 150mg | Sugar: 3g (natural sugars from raspberries) | Cholesterol: 0mg

CHILLED MANGO SOUP WITH MINT

This Chilled Mango Soup with Mint is a fresh and flavorful dessert that satisfies sweet cravings while adhering to the fatty liver diet guidelines. It is rich in vitamins and fiber, utilizing natural sugars from mangoes, enhanced with a hint of mint for a refreshing finish.

- **Prep Time:** 15 minutes
- **Cooking Time:** 0 minutes
- **Complexity:** Beginner
- **Servings:** 4
- **Ingredients:** 5

EQUIPMENT NEEDED: blender, measuring cups, spoons, serving bowls

TAGS: Whole Foods, Vegan, Gluten-Free, Dairy-Free, Low Glycemic, Heart-Healthy, High-fiber, Low Sodium, Low-fat, Low-calorie, Vitamin A rich, Vitamin C rich

INGREDIENT LIST:

- 2 large ripe mangoes, peeled and diced (about 2 cups, 500 ml)
- 1 cup coconut water (240 ml)
- Juice of 1 lime (about 2 tablespoons, 30 ml)
- 1 tablespoon chopped fresh mint, plus extra leaves for garnish (15 ml)
- 1 teaspoon freshly grated ginger (5 ml)

DIRECTIONS:

1. Place the diced mangoes, coconut water, lime juice, chopped mint, and grated ginger in a blender.
2. Blend until smooth and thoroughly combined.
3. Chill the mixture in the refrigerator for at least 2 hours, allowing the flavors to meld together.
4. Serve the chilled mango soup in bowls, garnished with additional mint leaves, for a touch of elegance and an extra burst of flavor.

NUTRITION INFORMATION: (APPROXIMATE VALUES PER SERVING): Calories: 120 | Protein: 1g | Carbohydrates: 30g | Sodium: 60mg | Fats: 0.5g | Potassium: 300mg | Sugar: 25g (natural sugars from mangoes) | Cholesterol: 0mg

FRESH BERRY SALAD WITH MINT

Enjoy a vibrant and nutritious dessert with this Fresh Berry Salad with Mint. Perfect for those following a fatty liver diet, this simple dish combines a variety of fresh berries with a hint of mint, providing a delicious way to satisfy your sweet tooth without added sugars.

Prep Time: 10 minutes | **Cooking Time:** 0 minutes | **Complexity:** Beginner | **Servings:** 4 | **Ingredients:** 4

EQUIPMENT NEEDED: bowl, knife, cutting board, spoons

TAGS: Whole Foods, Vegan, Gluten-Free, Dairy-Free, Sugar-Free, Low Glycemic, Heart-Healthy, High-fiber, Low Sodium, Low-fat, Low-calorie, Vitamin C rich

INGREDIENT LIST:

- 1 cup fresh strawberries, hulled and halved (150 g)
- 1 cup fresh blueberries (150 g)
- 1 cup fresh raspberries (125 g)
- 1/4 cup fresh mint leaves, finely chopped (15 g)

DIRECTIONS:

1. In a large mixing bowl, combine the strawberries, blueberries, and raspberries.
2. Gently toss the berries with the chopped mint leaves until evenly distributed.
3. Serve the berry salad immediately, or chill in the refrigerator for 30 minutes to enhance the mingling of flavors.

NUTRITION INFORMATION: (APPROXIMATE VALUES PER SERVING): Calories: 70 | Protein: 1.5g | Carbohydrates: 17g | Sodium: 5mg | Fats: 0.5g | Potassium: 130mg | Sugar: 11g | Cholesterol: 0mg

DATE AND NUT TRUFFLES

Indulge in these Date and Nut Truffles, a delightful treat crafted to align with a fatty liver diet. Made with whole ingredients, these truffles are naturally sweetened with dates and enriched with nuts, offering a guilt-free way to satisfy your sweet cravings.

Prep Time: 15 minutes | **Cooking Time:** 0 minutes | **Complexity:** Beginner | **Servings:** 8 | **Ingredients:** 5

EQUIPMENT NEEDED: food processor, bowl, tray, spoons

TAGS: Whole Foods, Vegan, Gluten-Free, Dairy-Free, Sugar-Free, Low Glycemic, Heart-Healthy, High-protein, High-fiber, Low Sodium, Low-fat, Low-calorie, Vitamin E rich

INGREDIENT LIST:

- 1 cup pitted Medjool dates (200 g)
- 1/2 cup raw almonds (75 g)
- 1/2 cup raw walnuts (75 g)
- 1/4 cup unsweetened cocoa powder (30 g)
- 1/4 teaspoon sea salt (1.5 g)

DIRECTIONS:

1. Place the almonds and walnuts in a food processor and pulse until finely ground.
2. Add the pitted dates, cocoa powder, and sea salt to the food processor. Process until the mixture begins to stick together and form a dough-like consistency.
3. Scoop out tablespoon-sized portions of the mixture and roll them into balls using your hands.
4. Place the truffles on a tray lined with parchment paper. Refrigerate for at least 30 minutes to set.
5. Serve chilled or store in an airtight container in the refrigerator for up to one week.

NUTRITION INFORMATION: (APPROXIMATE VALUES PER SERVING): Calories: 180 | Protein: 4g | Carbohydrates: 21g | Sodium: 75mg | Fats: 11g | Potassium: 300mg | Sugar: 15g | Cholesterol: 0mg

COCONUT AND LIME RICE PUDDING

Delight in this Coconut and Lime Rice Pudding, a creamy and tangy dessert that adheres strictly to fatty liver diet recommendations. This comforting dish combines the rich flavor of coconut with a zest of lime, offering a refreshing twist to traditional rice pudding.

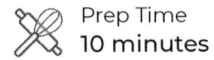

Prep Time: 10 minutes
Cooking Time: 30 minutes
Complexity: Beginner
Servings: 4
Ingredients: 7

EQUIPMENT NEEDED: saucepan, whisk, bowl, spoon
TAGS: Whole Foods, Vegan, Gluten-Free, Dairy-Free, Sugar-Free, Low Glycemic, Heart-Healthy, High-fiber, Low Sodium, Low-fat

INGREDIENT LIST:

- 1 cup brown rice, cooked (190 g)
- 2 cups unsweetened coconut milk (480 ml)
- 1/4 cup fresh lime juice (60 ml)
- Zest of one lime
- 2 tablespoons chia seeds (30 g)
- 1/4 cup shredded unsweetened coconut (20 g)
- 1 tablespoon erythritol (optional, for added sweetness) (12.5 g)

DIRECTIONS:

1. In a medium saucepan, combine the cooked brown rice and coconut milk. Bring to a simmer over medium heat.
2. Once simmering, reduce the heat to low and cook for about 20 minutes, stirring occasionally, until the mixture thickens and the rice becomes very tender.
3. Stir in the lime juice, lime zest, chia seeds, and shredded coconut. Continue to cook for an additional 10 minutes, allowing the flavors to meld together and the pudding to thicken further.
4. Remove from heat and stir in erythritol if using, for a touch of sweetness.
5. Divide the pudding into serving bowls. It can be served warm or chilled in the refrigerator for a couple of hours to serve cold.
6. Garnish with a sprinkle of lime zest and a few coconut shreds before serving.

NUTRITION INFORMATION: (APPROXIMATE VALUES PER SERVING): Calories: 215 | Protein: 3g | Carbohydrates: 28g | Sodium: 30mg | Fats: 11g | Potassium: 200mg | Sugar: 1g | Cholesterol: 0mg

BAKED PEACHES WITH CRUSHED ALMONDS

Indulge in a delightful and nutritious dessert of Baked Peaches with Crushed Almonds. This easy-to-prepare treat combines the natural sweetness of peaches with the crunchy texture of almonds, making it a perfect dish to satisfy your sweet cravings without straying from a fatty liver diet.

Prep Time: 10 minutes
Cooking Time: 25 minutes
Complexity: Beginner
Servings: 4
Ingredients: 5

EQUIPMENT NEEDED: baking dish, bowl, spoon, knife
TAGS: Whole Foods, Vegetarian, Gluten-Free, Dairy-Free, Low Glycemic, Heart-Healthy, High-Fiber, Low Sodium, Low-Fat, Vitamin A rich, Vitamin C rich

INGREDIENT LIST:

- 4 large peaches, halved and pitted (4 peaches)
- 1/2 cup crushed almonds (60 g)
- 1/4 teaspoon ground cinnamon (0.5 g)
- 1 tablespoon honey, optional (for extra sweetness if desired) (15 ml)
- Fresh mint leaves for garnish

DIRECTIONS:

1. Preheat your oven to 375 degrees Fahrenheit (190 degrees Celsius). Place the peach halves, cut side up, in a baking dish.
2. In a small bowl, mix the crushed almonds with cinnamon and sprinkle this mixture over the peach halves.
3. Drizzle a small amount of honey over each peach half if using.
4. Bake in the preheated oven for 25 minutes or until the peaches are tender and the topping is golden brown.
5. Remove from the oven and allow to cool slightly before serving.
6. Garnish with fresh mint leaves to enhance the flavor and presentation.

NUTRITION INFORMATION: (APPROXIMATE VALUES PER SERVING): Calories: 150 | Protein: 4g | Carbohydrates: 21g | Sodium: 0mg | Fats: 7g | Potassium: 410mg | Sugar: 15g | Cholesterol: 0mg

ZUCCHINI AND CHOCOLATE CHIP BREAD (SUGAR-FREE)

Savor a slice of Zucchini and Chocolate Chip Bread, a delectable, sugar-free treat that blends the moistness of zucchini with the rich taste of chocolate chips. This healthy dessert option aligns perfectly with a fatty liver diet, providing a satisfying sweet without any added sugars.

Prep Time: 15 minutes
Cooking Time: 50 minutes
Complexity: Beginner
Servings: 8
Ingredients: 10

EQUIPMENT NEEDED: bowl, whisk, spatula, loaf pan, measuring cups, measuring spoons

TAGS: Whole Foods, Vegetarian, Gluten-Free, Sugar-Free, High-Fiber, Low Sodium, Low Fat, Vitamin C rich

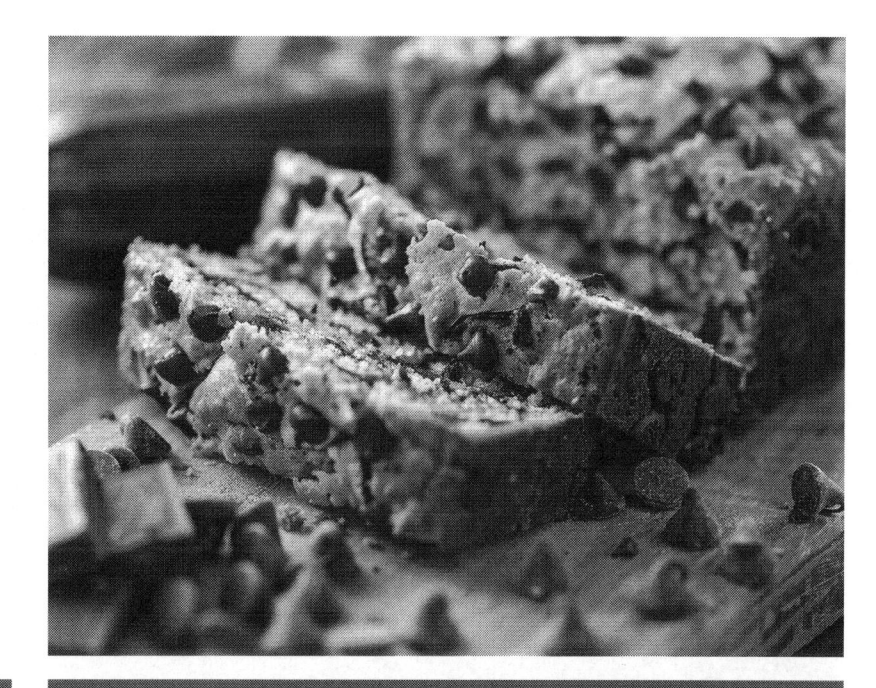

INGREDIENT LIST:

- 4 monkfish fillets (6 ounces each) (170 g each)
- 1 tablespoon olive oil (15 ml)
- 1 teaspoon ground turmeric (5 ml)
- 1 teaspoon ground cumin (5 ml)
- 1 teaspoon ground coriander (5 ml)
- 1 cup red lentils, rinsed (190 g)
- 4 cups low-sodium vegetable broth (960 ml)
- 1 large onion, finely chopped (about 150 g)
- 2 cloves garlic, minced (approx. 6 g)
- 1 tablespoon grated ginger (15 g)
- 1 teaspoon garam masala (5 ml)
- Salt and pepper to taste (minimal)

DIRECTIONS:

1. Heat olive oil in a sauté pan over medium heat. Add turmeric, cumin, and coriander; stir for 30 seconds to release the flavors.
2. Add monkfish fillets to the pan, season with salt and pepper, and cook for 4-5 minutes on each side until the fish is cooked through and lightly browned. Remove and set aside.
3. In the same pan, add more oil if needed, and sauté onion, garlic, and ginger until onion is translucent, about 5 minutes.
4. Add lentils and vegetable broth to the pan. Bring to a boil, then reduce heat and simmer for 20-25 minutes, or until lentils are soft and the mixture has thickened.
5. Stir in garam masala and season with salt and pepper to taste.
6. Serve the spiced monkfish over a bed of creamy lentil dal.

NUTRITION INFORMATION: (APPROXIMATE VALUES PER SERVING): Calories: 180 | Protein: 4g | Carbohydrates: 27g | Sodium: 160mg | Fats: 7g | Potassium: 125mg | Sugar: 2g | Cholesterol: 20mg

SUGAR-FREE ALMOND BUTTER BROWNIES

Indulge in these rich, fudgy, Sugar-Free Almond Butter Brownies, a delightful treat that satisfies your sweet tooth while adhering to a fatty liver diet. Made with healthful ingredients, these brownies offer a guilt-free dessert option perfect for those managing their sugar intake.

Prep Time: 10 minutes
Cooking Time: 25 minutes
Complexity: Beginner
Servings: 12
Ingredients: 8

EQUIPMENT NEEDED: bowl, spatula, baking pan, oven, measuring cups, measuring spoons

TAGS: Sugar-Free, Gluten-Free, Vegetarian, High-Fiber, Low Sodium, Whole Foods, Low Glycemic, Heart-Healthy, High Protein

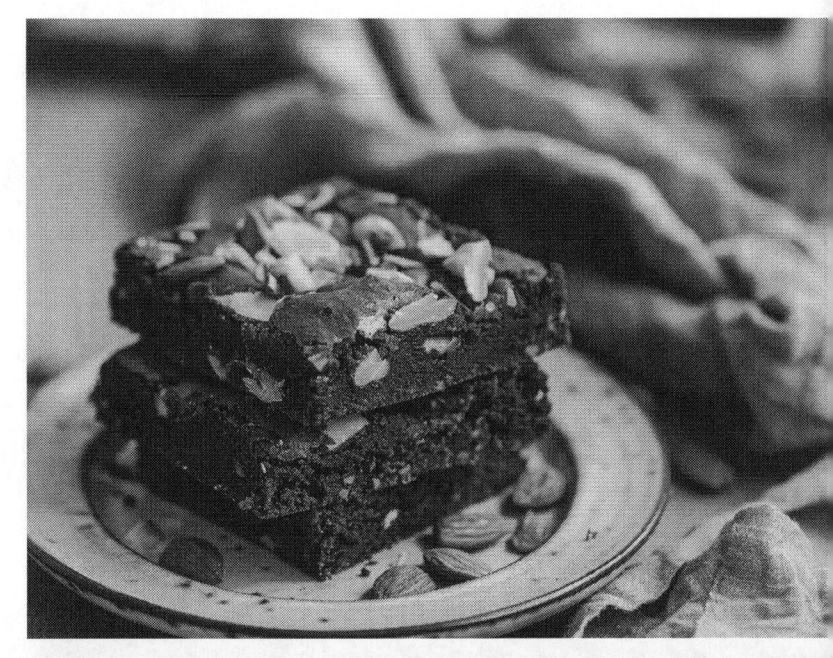

INGREDIENT LIST:

- 1 cup natural almond butter (smooth) (240 g)
- 1/3 cup granulated monk fruit sweetener (80 ml)
- 1/4 cup unsweetened cocoa powder (30 g)
- 1/2 teaspoon baking soda (2.5 g)
- 1/4 teaspoon salt (1.25 g)
- 2 large eggs (substitute with flax eggs for vegan option) (100 g)
- 1 teaspoon vanilla extract (5 ml)
- 1/2 cup unsweetened almond milk (120 ml)
- Optional: 1/2 cup sugar-free dark chocolate chips (85 g) for extra richness

DIRECTIONS:

1. Preheat the oven to 350°F (175°C). Grease or line an 8-inch square baking pan with parchment paper.
2. In a large mixing bowl, combine the almond butter and monk fruit sweetener. Stir until well blended.
3. Add the cocoa powder, baking soda, and salt. Mix thoroughly to eliminate any lumps.
4. Beat in the eggs, one at a time, then stir in the vanilla extract and almond milk until the mixture is smooth.
5. If using, fold in the sugar-free dark chocolate chips.
6. Pour the batter into the prepared baking pan, spreading it evenly.
7. Bake in the preheated oven for about 25 minutes or until a toothpick inserted into the center comes out mostly clean.
8. Allow the brownies to cool in the pan for at least 10 minutes before slicing them into squares.

NUTRITION INFORMATION: (APPROXIMATE VALUES PER SERVING): Calories: 160 | Protein: 6g | Carbohydrates: 8g | Sodium: 90mg | Fats: 12g | Potassium: 200mg | Sugar: 1g | Cholesterol: 30mg

CHAPTER 11: HYDRATING DRINKS AND SMOOTHIES

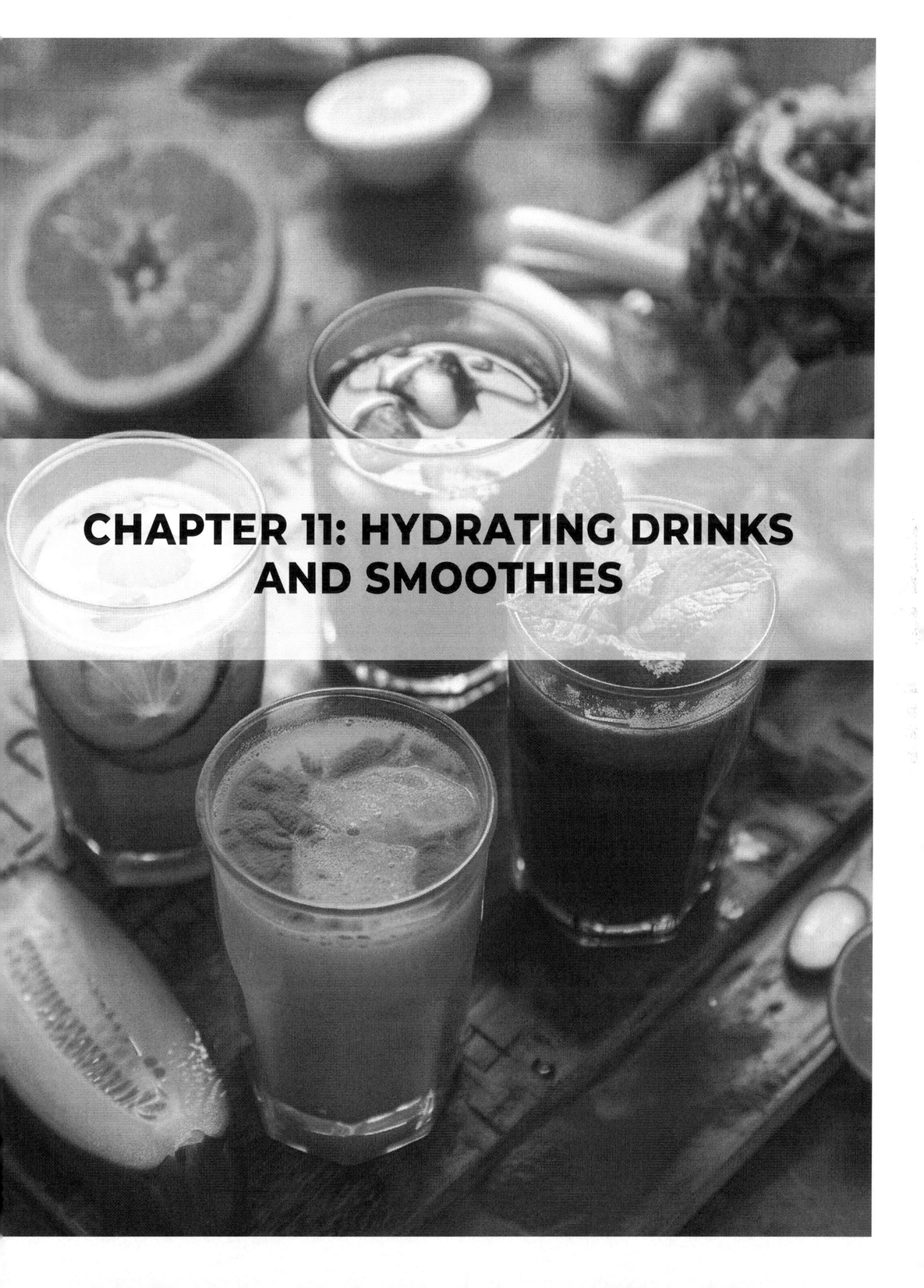

CARROT, ORANGE, AND GINGER IMMUNE BOOSTER

Energize your day with this vibrant Carrot, Orange, and Ginger Immune Booster. Packed with vitamin C, fiber, and essential nutrients, this refreshing drink is perfect for supporting liver health and boosting your immune system.

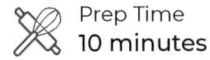

Prep Time: 10 minutes
Cooking Time: 0 minutes
Complexity: Beginner
Servings: 2
Ingredients: 5

EQUIPMENT NEEDED: juicer, knife, cutting board, measuring spoons, serving glasses

TAGS: Whole Foods, Vegan, Gluten-Free, Low Glycemic, Heart-Healthy, High-Fiber, Low Sodium, Low Fat, Sugar-Free, Vitamin A Rich, Vitamin C Rich, Vitamin E Rich

INGREDIENT LIST:

- 4 large carrots, peeled and chopped (400 g)
- 2 large oranges, peeled and quartered (300 g)
- 1 inch fresh ginger, peeled (2.5 cm)
- 1 tablespoon lemon juice (15 ml)
- Ice cubes (optional)

DIRECTIONS:

1. Prepare all ingredients: peel and chop the carrots, peel and quarter the oranges, and peel the ginger.
2. Place carrots, oranges, and ginger through the juicer.
3. Stir in the lemon juice into the freshly extracted juice to enhance flavor and add an extra boost of vitamin C.
4. Serve immediately over ice if desired for a refreshing and invigorating drink.

NUTRITION INFORMATION: (APPROXIMATE VALUES PER SERVING): Calories: 95 | Protein: 2g | Carbohydrates: 22g | Sodium: 60mg | Fats: 0.5g | Potassium: 450mg | Sugar: 15g | Cholesterol: 0mg

CUCUMBER, CELERY, AND LIME HYDRATION DRINK

Replenish your body with this ultra-refreshing Cucumber, Celery, and Lime Hydration Drink. Designed to hydrate and nourish, this easy-to-make beverage is perfect for liver health and overall wellness.

Prep Time: 5 minutes
Cooking Time: 0 minutes
Complexity: Beginner
Servings: 2
Ingredients: 4

EQUIPMENT NEEDED: Replenish your body with this ultra-refreshing Cucumber, Celery, and Lime Hydration Drink. Designed to hydrate and nourish, this easy-to-make beverage is perfect for liver health and overall wellness.

TAGS: Whole Foods, Vegan, Gluten-Free, Low Glycemic, Heart-Healthy, High-Fiber, Low Sodium, Low Fat, Sugar-Free, Vitamin C Rich

INGREDIENT LIST:

- 1 large cucumber, chopped (about 300 g)
- 2 stalks celery, chopped (about 100 g)
- Juice of 2 limes (about 60 ml)
- 1 cup water (240 ml)
- Ice cubes (optional for serving)

DIRECTIONS:

1. Wash the cucumber and celery thoroughly. Chop them into manageable pieces for blending.
2. Combine the chopped cucumber, celery, lime juice, and water in a blender.
3. Blend on high until smooth.
4. Strain the mixture using a fine mesh strainer into a pitcher to remove the pulp, extracting as much liquid as possible.
5. Serve the strained juice over ice if desired for a chilled and more refreshing experience.

NUTRITION INFORMATION: (APPROXIMATE VALUES PER SERVING): Calories: 35 | Protein: 1g | Carbohydrates: 8g | Sodium: 40mg | Fats: 0g | Potassium: 270mg | Sugar: 4g | Cholesterol: 0mg

RASPBERRY, LIME, AND COCONUT WATER SLUSHIE

Quench your thirst and boost your nutrient intake with this Raspberry, Lime, and Coconut Water Slushie. Perfect for hydration and rich in antioxidants, this slushie is a delightful treat on a hot day or after a workout.

- **Prep Time:** 5 minutes
- **Cooking Time:** 0 minutes
- **Complexity:** Beginner
- **Servings:** 2
- **Ingredients:** 4

EQUIPMENT NEEDED: blender, measuring cups, knife

TAGS: Whole Foods, Vegan, Gluten-Free, Low Glycemic, Heart-Healthy, High-Fiber, Low Sodium, Low Fat, Sugar-Free, Vitamin C Rich

INGREDIENT LIST:

- 1 cup fresh raspberries (about 125g)
- Juice of 1 lime (about 2 tablespoons or 30 ml)
- 2 cups coconut water (480 ml)
- 1 cup ice cubes (about 120g)

DIRECTIONS:

1. Rinse the raspberries under cold water.
2. In a blender, combine the fresh raspberries, freshly squeezed lime juice, coconut water, and ice cubes.
3. Blend on high until the mixture reaches a slushie consistency.
4. Pour into glasses and serve immediately for the best flavor and texture.

NUTRITION INFORMATION: (APPROXIMATE VALUES PER SERVING): Calories: 90 | Protein: 2g | Carbohydrates: 22g | Sodium: 252mg | Fats: 1g | Potassium: 667mg | Sugar: 15g | Cholesterol: 0mg

GREEN TEA INFUSION WITH MINT AND LEMON

This refreshing Green Tea Infusion with Mint and Lemon is the perfect drink to aid digestion and boost your antioxidant intake. Ideal for hydration, it helps maintain liver health and manages energy levels throughout the day.

- **Prep Time:** 5 minutes
- **Cooking Time:** 5 minutes
- **Complexity:** Beginner
- **Servings:** 2
- **Ingredients:** 4

EQUIPMENT NEEDED: teapot, measuring cups, knife, cutting board

TAGS: Whole Foods, Vegan, Gluten-Free, Low Glycemic, Heart-Healthy, Low Sodium, Low Fat, Sugar-Free, High Antioxidants, Vitamin C rich

INGREDIENT LIST:

- 2 teaspoons green tea leaves (or 2 green tea bags)
- 12 fresh mint leaves
- 1 organic lemon, juiced (about 3 tablespoons or 45 ml)
- 4 cups boiling water (960 ml)

DIRECTIONS:

1. Boil 4 cups of water in a kettle.
2. Place the green tea leaves or tea bags and fresh mint leaves into a teapot.
3. Pour the boiling water over the tea and mint leaves and allow it to steep for about 3-5 minutes.
4. Strain the infusion into cups or a large pitcher.
5. Stir in the fresh lemon juice.
6. Serve the tea warm or chill it in the refrigerator to serve cold over ice.

NUTRITION INFORMATION: (APPROXIMATE VALUES PER SERVING): Calories: 10 | Protein: 0g | Carbohydrates: 3g | Sodium: 0mg | Fats: 0g | Potassium: 49mg | Sugar: 1g | Cholesterol: 0mg

PINEAPPLE AND FRESH TURMERIC DIGESTIVE AID

This Pineapple and Fresh Turmeric Digestive Aid is a vibrant drink packed with anti-inflammatory benefits and enzymes to help soothe the digestive system, making it a perfect choice for those managing fatty liver disease.

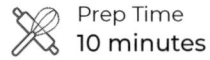

Prep Time: 10 minutes
Cooking Time: 0 minutes
Complexity: Beginner
Servings: 2
Ingredients: 5

EQUIPMENT NEEDED: blender, knife, cutting board, measuring cups

TAGS: Whole Foods, Vegan, Gluten-Free, Low Glycemic, Heart-Healthy, Low Sodium, High Fiber, Low Fat, Sugar-Free, Vitamin C rich, Anti-Inflammatory

INGREDIENT LIST:

- 2 cups fresh pineapple, cubed (about 300g)
- 1 inch fresh turmeric root, peeled (about 2.5 cm)
- 1 tablespoon fresh lime juice (about 15 ml)
- 1 cup coconut water (240 ml)
- 1/2 cup ice cubes (about 120 ml)

DIRECTIONS:

1. Prepare the pineapple by peeling, coring, and cutting it into cubes.
2. Peel the fresh turmeric root using a small knife or spoon.
3. Place the pineapple cubes, fresh turmeric, lime juice, coconut water, and ice cubes into a blender.
4. Blend on high speed until smooth and frothy.
5. Pour into glasses and serve immediately for the freshest taste and most digestive benefits.

NUTRITION INFORMATION: (APPROXIMATE VALUES PER SERVING): Calories: 95 | Protein: 1g | Carbohydrates: 23g | Sodium: 60mg | Fats: 0.5g | Potassium: 300mg | Sugar: 17g | Cholesterol: 0mg

MATCHA AND SPIRULINA ENERGY DRINK

Revitalize your body with this Matcha and Spirulina Energy Drink, a powerhouse blend that combines the antioxidant benefits of matcha with the nutritional prowess of spirulina. This drink is perfect for boosting energy levels while supporting liver health.

Prep Time: 5 minutes
Cooking Time: 0 minutes
Complexity: Beginner
Servings: 1
Ingredients: 5

EQUIPMENT NEEDED: blender, measuring spoons, glass

TAGS: Whole Foods, Vegan, Gluten-Free, Low Glycemic, Heart-Healthy, Low Sodium, High Protein, High Fiber, Low Fat, Sugar-Free, Vitamin C rich, Antioxidant-rich

INGREDIENT LIST:

- 1 teaspoon matcha green tea powder (5 ml)
- 1 teaspoon spirulina powder (5 ml)
- 1 cup unsweetened almond milk (240 ml)
- 1 tablespoon chia seeds (15 ml)
- Ice cubes (as needed)

DIRECTIONS:

1. Add the matcha green tea powder and spirulina powder to the blender.
2. Pour in the unsweetened almond milk and add the chia seeds.
3. Add a handful of ice cubes to achieve a chilled, refreshing texture.
4. Blend on high until the mixture is smooth and the chia seeds are well incorporated.
5. Pour the drink into a glass and enjoy it immediately for maximum freshness and effectiveness.

NUTRITION INFORMATION: (APPROXIMATE VALUES PER SERVING): Calories: 100 | Protein: 4g | Carbohydrates: 9g | Sodium: 180mg | Fats: 5g | Potassium: 135mg | Sugar: 0g | Cholesterol: 0mg

SOOTHING CHAMOMILE AND LAVENDER TEA

Unwind with this calming, Soothing Chamomile and Lavender Tea, crafted to ease stress and support liver health. Ideal for relaxation, this herbal infusion blends the gentle qualities of chamomile with the soothing aroma of lavender, promoting a sense of well-being.

- **Prep Time:** 5 minutes
- **Cooking Time:** 10 minutes
- **Complexity:** Beginner
- **Servings:** 1
- **Ingredients:** 4

EQUIPMENT NEEDED: kettle, tea infuser or teapot, cup

TAGS: Zero Sugar, Whole Foods, Vegan, Gluten-Free, Low Glycemic, Heart-Healthy, Vegetarian, Dairy-Free, Low Sodium, Low Fat, Low Calorie, Vitamin C rich, Antioxidant-rich

INGREDIENT LIST:

- 1 tablespoon dried chamomile flowers (15 ml)
- 1 teaspoon dried lavender flowers (5 ml)
- 1 cup of boiling water (240 ml)
- Optional: a slice of lemon for added vitamin C and flavor

DIRECTIONS:

1. Boil water in a kettle.
2. Place the dried chamomile and lavender flowers in a tea infuser or directly into a teapot.
3. Pour the boiling water over the chamomile and lavender flowers. Allow to steep for about 8-10 minutes, depending on desired strength.
4. Remove the infuser or strain the tea to remove the flowers.
5. Optional: Add a slice of lemon to the brewed tea for a refreshing twist and a boost of vitamin C.
6. Serve the tea warm and enjoy the relaxing benefits.

NUTRITION INFORMATION: (APPROXIMATE VALUES PER SERVING): Calories: 10 | Protein: 0g | Carbohydrates: 0g | Sodium: 0mg | Fats: 0g | Potassium: 9mg | Sugar: 0g | Cholesterol: 0mg

MANGO, KIWI, AND SPINACH SMOOTHIE

Enjoy the refreshing taste and nutritional benefits of this Mango, Kiwi, and Spinach Smoothie. This vibrant blend is perfect for supporting liver health, packed with vitamin-rich fruits and fiber-dense spinach to keep you hydrated and nourished.

- **Prep Time:** 10 minutes
- **Cooking Time:** 0 minutes
- **Complexity:** Beginner
- **Servings:** 2
- **Ingredients:** 5

EQUIPMENT NEEDED: blender, measuring cups, knife

TAGS: Whole Foods, Vegan, Gluten-Free, Dairy-Free, Low Glycemic, Heart-Healthy, High Fiber, Low Sodium, Low Fat, Low Calorie, Vitamin A rich, Vitamin C rich, Vegetarian

INGREDIENT LIST:

- 1 ripe mango, peeled and cubed (about 200 g)
- 2 kiwis, peeled and sliced (about 150 g)
- 2 cups fresh spinach leaves (60 g)
- 1 tablespoon ground flaxseed (15 ml) [for added fiber and omega-3s]
- 1 cup unsweetened almond milk (240 ml)

DIRECTIONS:

1. Prepare the fruits: Peel and cube the mango, and peel and slice the kiwis.
2. Place the mango, kiwi slices, fresh spinach, ground flaxseed, and unsweetened almond milk into a blender.
3. Blend on high until smooth, ensuring all the spinach leaves are fully incorporated, and the smoothie achieves a creamy consistency.
4. Pour into glasses and serve immediately to enjoy its full flavor and nutrient content.

NUTRITION INFORMATION: (APPROXIMATE VALUES PER SERVING): Calories: 180 | Protein: 3g | Carbohydrates: 35g | Sodium: 55mg | Fats: 3g | Potassium: 490mg | Sugar: 25g | Cholesterol: 0mg

TURMERIC AND PINEAPPLE ANTI-INFLAMMATORY SMOOTHIE

Jumpstart your day with this vibrant Turmeric and Pineapple Anti-Inflammatory Smoothie, packed with nutrients to support liver health and reduce inflammation. This refreshing blend of pineapple, turmeric, and ginger not only tastes delicious but also delivers a potent dose of antioxidants.

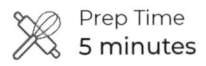

Prep Time: 5 minutes
Cooking Time: 0 minutes
Complexity: Beginner
Servings: 2
Ingredients: 6

EQUIPMENT NEEDED: blender, measuring cups, spoons

TAGS: Whole Foods, Vegan, Gluten-Free, Dairy-Free, Low Glycemic, Heart-Healthy, High Fiber, Low Sodium, Low Fat, Low Calorie, Vitamin C rich, Anti-inflammatory

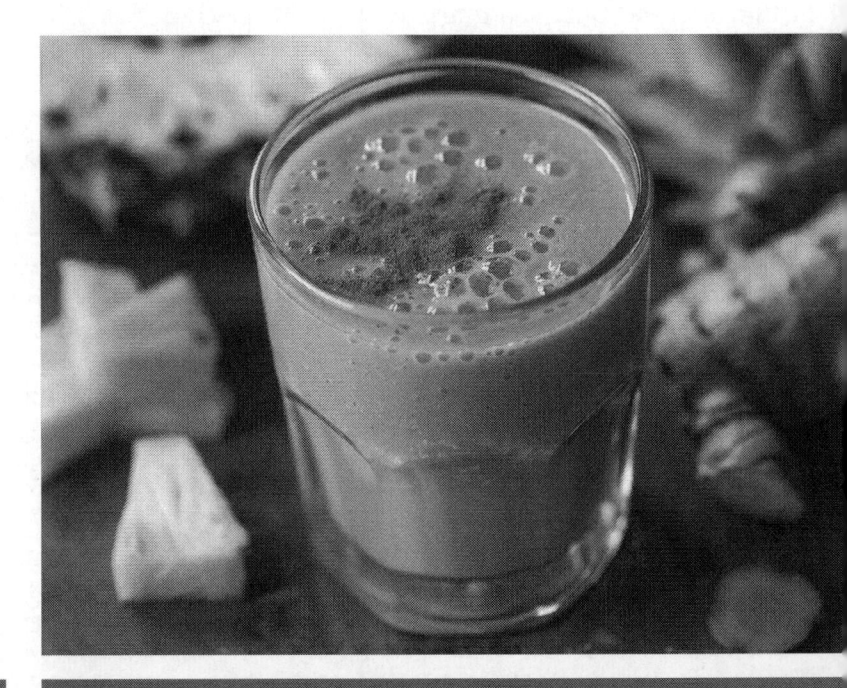

INGREDIENT LIST:

- 1 cup fresh pineapple chunks (165 g)
- 1 banana, sliced (~ 100 g)
- 1/2 inch fresh turmeric root, peeled and chopped (about 3 g)
- 1/2 inch fresh ginger root, peeled and chopped (about 3 g)
- 1 tablespoon chia seeds (15 ml)
- 1 cup unsweetened almond milk (240 ml)

DIRECTIONS:

1. Prepare all ingredients: Peel and chop the fresh turmeric and ginger root. Slice the banana and measure out the pineapple chunks.
2. Place the pineapple, banana, turmeric, ginger, chia seeds, and almond milk in a blender.
3. Blend on high until smooth and creamy, ensuring that the turmeric and ginger are well incorporated.
4. Pour the smoothie into glasses and serve immediately for maximum freshness and flavor.

NUTRITION INFORMATION: (APPROXIMATE VALUES PER SERVING): Calories: 150 | Protein: 3g | Carbohydrates: 25g | Sodium: 40mg | Fats: 4g | Potassium: 422mg | Sugar: 14g | Cholesterol: 0mg

PEAR AND GINGER SOOTHER

A soothing and refreshing drink, this Pear and Ginger Soother combines the natural sweetness of ripe pears with the zesty kick of ginger, making it a perfect beverage to aid digestion and enhance hydration.

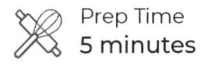

Prep Time: 5 minutes
Cooking Time: 0 minutes
Complexity: Beginner
Servings: 2
Ingredients: 4

EQUIPMENT NEEDED: blender, knife, measuring cups

TAGS: Whole Foods, Vegan, Gluten-Free, Dairy-Free, Low Glycemic, Heart-Healthy, High Fiber, Low Sodium, Low Fat, Low Calorie, Vitamin C rich, Vegetarian

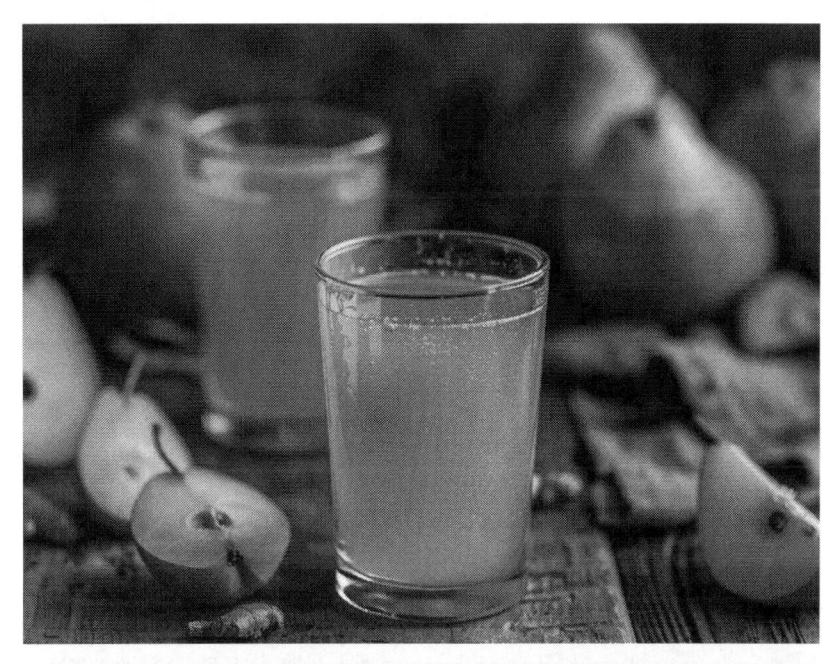

INGREDIENT LIST:

- 2 ripe pears, cored and chopped (about 350 g)
- 1-inch piece of fresh ginger, peeled and minced (about 2.5 cm)
- Juice of 1 lemon (about 45 ml)
- 1 cup cold water (240 ml)

DIRECTIONS:

1. Prepare the ingredients: Core and chop the pears; peel and finely mince the ginger.
2. Place the chopped pears, minced ginger, freshly squeezed lemon juice, and cold water into a blender.
3. Blend on high until the mixture is smooth and fully combined.
4. Strain through a fine mesh sieve into glasses to remove any pulp or ginger fibers, if desired, for a smoother texture.
5. Serve immediately, garnished with a slice of lemon or a sprig of mint for an extra touch of freshness.

NUTRITION INFORMATION: (APPROXIMATE VALUES PER SERVING): Calories: 120 | Protein: 1g | Carbohydrates: 31g | Sodium: 10mg | Fats: 0g | Potassium: 212mg | Sugar: 20g | Cholesterol: 0mg

CHAPTER 12: COMPREHENSIVE 30-DAY MEAL PLAN

DAY	BREAKFAST	LUNCH	DINNER	SUPPER	TOTAL KCAL
1	Spiced Pumpkin Porridge	Quinoa Tabbouleh with Chickpeas	Stir-Fried Kale and Quinoa	Baked Cod Fish Sticks with Yogurt Dill Sauce	870
2	Cottage Cheese Pancakes with Blueberries	Garlic Roasted Trout with Brussels Sprouts	Pumpkin and Black Bean Casserole	Smoked Salmon and Cream Cheese Cucumber Rolls	810
3	Vegetable Hash with Poached Egg	Hearty Minestrone Soup with Whole Wheat Pasta	Roasted Cauliflower and Chickpea Tacos	Cucumber Boats with Spicy Shrimp Salad	890
4	Vegan Tofu Scramble with Spinach and Tomatoes	Vegan Buddha Bowl with Spiced Chickpeas	Creamy Broccoli and Spinach Soup	Roasted Brussels Sprouts with Lemon Dip	730
5	Walnut and Pear Oat Bake	Carrot and Ginger Purée Soup	Blackened Catfish with Collard Greens	Ricotta and Berry Stuffed Celery	860
6	Salmon and Avocado Toast	Spinach and Mushroom Polenta Stacks	Citrus Roasted Turkey Breast	Zucchini and Herb Fritters	1150
7	Pear and Walnut Oatmeal	Grilled Haddock with Olive Tapenade	Sautéed Brussels Sprouts with Crispy Tofu	Tahini and Cocoa Energy Bites	925
8	Quinoa and Apple Breakfast Bowl	Tuna and White Bean Salad	Vegetable and Tofu Pad Thai	Pumpkin Hummus with Whole Grain Pita Chips	1050
9	Smoked Salmon and Avocado Toast	Roasted Vegetable and Farro Bowl	Stuffed Portobello Mushrooms with Spinach and Feta	Kale and Apple Chips	940
10	Grilled Chicken and Avocado Wrap	Cod in Parsley Cream Sauce	Hearty Minestrone Soup with Whole Wheat Pasta	Air-Fried Spiced Carrot Chips	950
11	Pear and Walnut Oatmeal	Grilled Haddock with Olive Tapenade	Sautéed Brussels Sprouts with Crispy Tofu	Air-Fried Spiced Carrot Chips	825

DAY	BREAKFAST	LUNCH	DINNER	SUPPER	TOTAL KCAL
12	Walnut and Pear Oat Bake	Garlic Roasted Trout with Brussels Sprouts	Blackened Catfish with Collard Greens	Zucchini and Herb Fritters	1045
13	Vegetable Hash with Poached Egg	Vegan Buddha Bowl with Spiced Chickpeas	Vegetable and Tofu Pad Thai	Pumpkin Hummus with Whole Grain Pita Chips	955
14	Spiced Pumpkin Porridge	Cod in Parsley Cream Sauce	Stir-Fried Kale and Quinoa	Smoked Salmon and Cream Cheese Cucumber Rolls	890
15	Quinoa and Apple Breakfast Bowl	Hearty Minestrone Soup with Whole Wheat Pasta	Creamy Broccoli and Spinach Soup	Ricotta and Berry Stuffed Celery	865
16	Cottage Cheese Pancakes with Blueberries	Tuna and White Bean Salad	Citrus Roasted Turkey Breast	Cucumber Boats with Spicy Shrimp Salad	1020
17	Salmon and Avocado Toast	Roasted Vegetable and Farro Bowl	Roasted Cauliflower and Chickpea Tacos	Kale and Apple Chips	930
18	Smoked Salmon and Avocado Toast	Spinach and Mushroom Polenta Stacks	Pumpkin and Black Bean Casserole	Tahini and Cocoa Energy Bites	1050
19	Vegan Tofu Scramble with Spinach and Tomatoes	Carrot and Ginger Purée Soup	Stuffed Portobello Mushrooms with Spinach and Feta	Baked Cod Fish Sticks with Yogurt Dill Sauce	780
20	Grilled Chicken and Avocado Wrap	Quinoa Tabbouleh with Chickpeas	Hearty Minestrone Soup with Whole Wheat Pasta	Roasted Brussels Sprouts with Lemon Dip	1025
21	Spiced Pumpkin Porridge	Roasted Vegetable and Farro Bowl	Stir-Fried Kale and Quinoa	Smoked Salmon and Cream Cheese Cucumber Rolls	860
22	Walnut and Pear Oat Bake	Tuna and White Bean Salad	Blackened Catfish with Collard Greens	Air-Fried Spiced Carrot Chips	970
23	Cottage Cheese Pancakes with Blueberries	Vegan Buddha Bowl with Spiced Chickpeas	Creamy Broccoli and Spinach Soup	Zucchini and Herb Fritters	800

DAY	BREAKFAST	LUNCH	DINNER	SUPPER	TOTAL KCAL
24	Vegetable Hash with Poached Egg	Cod in Parsley Cream Sauce	Roasted Cauliflower and Chickpea Tacos	Pumpkin Hummus with Whole Grain Pita Chips	1050
25	Vegan Tofu Scramble with Spinach and Tomatoes	Spinach and Mushroom Polenta Stacks	Vegetable and Tofu Pad Thai	Ricotta and Berry Stuffed Celery	910
26	Pear and Walnut Oatmeal	Garlic Roasted Trout with Brussels Sprouts	Citrus Roasted Turkey Breast	Cucumber Boats with Spicy Shrimp Salad	990
27	Grilled Chicken and Avocado Wrap	Hearty Minestrone Soup with Whole Wheat Pasta	Sautéed Brussels Sprouts with Crispy Tofu	Kale and Apple Chips	935
28	Quinoa and Apple Breakfast Bowl	Carrot and Ginger Purée Soup	Pumpkin and Black Bean Casserole	Tahini and Cocoa Energy Bites	875
29	Smoked Salmon and Avocado Toast	Quinoa Tabbouleh with Chickpeas	Stuffed Portobello Mushrooms with Spinach and Feta	Baked Cod Fish Sticks with Yogurt Dill Sauce	1005
30	Salmon and Avocado Toast	Grilled Haddock with Olive Tapenade	Hearty Minestrone Soup with Whole Wheat Pasta	Roasted Brussels Sprouts with Lemon Dip	1010

TIPS FOR MEAL PREP AND STORAGE

Proper meal preparation and storage are crucial for maintaining the quality and nutritional value of food, especially when following a diet plan for conditions like fatty liver. Here are some practical tips to ensure that your meals remain delicious and nutritious throughout the week:

1. Plan Ahead

a. Make a Shopping List: Based on the meal plan, create a detailed shopping list. This helps in buying only what is necessary, reducing waste and ensuring you have all ingredients on hand.

b. Schedule Prep Time: Set aside specific times during the week for meal preparation. This could be a few hours on a weekend or smaller intervals on specific weekdays.

2. Batch Cooking

a. Cook in Bulk: Prepare large portions of versatile ingredients at the start of the week. Grains like quinoa or rice, proteins like chicken or tofu, and a variety of steamed or roasted vegetables can be mixed and matched throughout the week.

b. Use the Oven Wisely: Roast multiple types of vegetables or bake several chicken breasts simultaneously to save energy and time.

3. Efficient Storage

a. Use Appropriate Containers: Invest in high-quality airtight containers to store your prepped meals. Glass containers are preferable as they don't retain odors or stains and can go from fridge to microwave safely.

b. Label Your Containers: Mark containers with the date of preparation. This not only helps in tracking freshness but also in using the oldest meals first to avoid spoilage.

4. Portion Control

a. Pre-portion Meals: Divide cooked meals into individual portions before storing. This makes it easy to grab a meal on the go and helps in managing portion sizes.

b. Balance Each Meal: Ensure that each container has a good balance of carbohydrates, proteins, and fats to maintain a consistent intake of nutrients.

5. Optimize Refrigeration

a. Set the Right Temperature: Keep your refrigerator below 40°F (4°C). This helps in slowing down the growth of bacteria and preserves the freshness of your food.

b. Store Strategically: Place items that need more cooling, like dairy and raw meat, in the coldest part, usually at the back of the fridge, while cooked meals can be more accessible at the front.

6. Freezing for Longevity

a. Freeze Extra Portions: If you cook in very large batches, consider freezing part of it. Most cooked meals can be frozen for up to 3 months. Thaw in the fridge overnight before reheating.

b. Avoid Freezer Burn: Use freezer-safe containers or bags, and make sure to remove as much air as possible before sealing to prevent freezer burn.

7. Safe Reheating

a. Reheat Properly: Ensure that meals are reheated to 165°F (74°C) to kill any potential bacteria. Use a food thermometer to check temperatures.

b. Stir While Heating: When reheating food in a microwave, stir it midway to allow even heat distribution.

By following these tips, you can make meal preparation a convenient, health-supportive, and enjoyable part of your routine, ensuring that you stay on track with your diet for managing fatty liver and overall health.

CHAPTER 13: BEYOND DIET: A HOLISTIC APPROACH TO LIVER HEALTH

In managing fatty liver disease, diet plays a crucial role. However, a comprehensive approach to liver health extends beyond what we eat. This chapter will explore essential aspects of a holistic approach to managing liver health, including exercise, stress reduction, and emotional support.

EXERCISE RECOMMENDATIONS AND TIPS FOR GETTING STARTED

Regular physical activity is a cornerstone of good health and is particularly beneficial for those managing fatty liver disease. Exercise helps to decrease liver fat, enhance insulin sensitivity, and reduce inflammation. Here are some guidelines and tips for incorporating exercise into your routine:

Types of Exercise Beneficial for Liver Health:
- Aerobic Exercise: Activities like walking, jogging, cycling, and swimming increase your heart rate, improve circulation, and can significantly reduce liver fat.
- Resistance Training: Weight lifting or using resistance bands helps build muscle, boost metabolism, and improve glucose metabolism, all of which are beneficial for liver health.

Getting Started with an Exercise Routine:
- Consult with a Professional: Before starting any new exercise program, especially if you have underlying health issues, consult with a healthcare provider.
- Start Slow: Begin with low-intensity exercises, and gradually increase the intensity and duration as your fitness improves.
- Set Realistic Goals: Aim for at least 150 minutes of moderate-intensity aerobic activity or 75 minutes of vigorous aerobic activity per week, as recommended by health guidelines, but tailor this to your current fitness level.
- Stay Consistent: Consistency is key. Try to incorporate physical activity into your daily routine and set specific times for your workouts.

Tips for Staying Motivated:
- Track Your Progress: Use a journal or an app to keep track of your exercise routines and progress.
- Mix It Up: Vary your exercise routine to keep it interesting and cover different aspects of fitness, like flexibility, endurance, and strength.
- Find a Workout Buddy: Exercising with a friend can increase your motivation and make physical activity more enjoyable.

STRESS REDUCTION TECHNIQUES: MEDITATION, YOGA, AND MORE

Managing stress is vital in the fight against fatty liver disease. Chronic stress can exacerbate inflammation and worsen liver health. Integrating stress reduction techniques into your life can help mitigate these effects.

Meditation:

- Benefits: Meditation helps in reducing stress, improving emotional balance, and enhancing overall health. It can lower cortisol levels and reduce the inflammatory response.
- Getting Started: Begin with a few minutes of meditation daily, using apps or online videos for guided sessions.

Yoga:

- Benefits: Yoga combines physical postures, breathing exercises, and meditation. It not only reduces stress but also improves physical flexibility and strength.
- How to Practice: Join a yoga class suitable for your level or follow online tutorials at home. Start with basic poses and gradually move to more advanced poses.

Additional Techniques:

- Deep Breathing Exercises: Simple deep breathing can significantly lower stress levels and improve your sense of well-being.
- Progressive Muscle Relaxation: This involves tensing and then relaxing different muscle groups in your body, which can reduce stress and promote physical relaxation.

NAVIGATING EMOTIONAL EATING AND BUILDING A SUPPORT NETWORK

Emotional eating can be a significant barrier in managing diet-related diseases, including fatty liver. Recognizing the triggers and establishing a support network can help you make more mindful food choices.

Understanding Emotional Eating:

- Identify Triggers: Keep a food diary to note what you eat, when, and how you feel. Over time, patterns will emerge that identify the emotional triggers for overeating.
- Develop Healthy Responses: Once you recognize the triggers, you can work on developing healthier responses, such as going for a walk, practicing deep breathing, or meditating.

Building a Support Network:

- Seek Professional Help: A dietitian, therapist, or support group can provide guidance and support tailored to your needs.
- Engage Friends and Family: Educate them about your condition and how they can support you. Having family and friends as part of your support system can make managing your diet and lifestyle changes more manageable.
- Connect with Others: Consider joining online forums or local support groups where you can connect with others facing similar challenges.

In conclusion, managing fatty liver disease is a multifaceted journey that involves more than just dietary adjustments. Incorporating regular exercise, reducing stress, navigating emotional eating, and building a strong support network are all crucial steps in maintaining optimal liver health and overall well-being. By adopting a holistic approach, you can effectively manage the symptoms of fatty liver disease and enhance your quality of life.

CHAPTER 14: NAVIGATING CHALLENGES AND MAINTAINING PROGRESS

Adopting and maintaining a healthy lifestyle, especially when managing conditions like fatty liver, can present various challenges. This chapter offers practical advice on adapting recipes to meet different dietary needs, overcoming common obstacles, and staying motivated throughout your health journey.

HOW TO ADAPT RECIPES FOR DIFFERENT DIETARY NEEDS (VEGAN, GLUTEN-FREE, ETC.)

Flexibility in your diet is crucial, especially when dietary restrictions or preferences are in play. Here are tips on how to modify recipes to suit various needs:

Vegan Adaptations:

- Proteins: Replace animal proteins with plant-based alternatives like lentils, chickpeas, tofu, and tempeh.
- Dairy: Use plant milk (almond, soy, oat) and vegan cheeses or yogurts. Coconut cream can substitute for heavy creams.
- Eggs: In baking, use flaxseeds or chia seeds mixed with water, mashed bananas, or commercial egg replacers.

Gluten-Free Adjustments:

- Flours: Substitute wheat flour with almond, oat, rice, or chickpea flour.
- Thickeners: Use cornstarch or arrowroot instead of flour for thickening sauces or gravies.
- Pasta and Breads: Opt for gluten-free alternatives available in most supermarkets; ensure they are also low in sugars and unhealthy fats.

Low-Carb Options:

- Sugars: Replace sugars with natural sweeteners like stevia or use pureed fruits to add sweetness.
- Grains: Substitute grains with cauliflower rice, zucchini noodles, or use lower-carb grains like quinoa or bulgur.

OVERCOMING COMMON OBSTACLES IN YOUR DIET AND LIFESTYLE CHANGES

Changing one's diet and lifestyle is no small feat. Here are common obstacles and ways to overcome them:

Time Constraints:

- Meal Prepping: Cook meals in bulk over the weekend or when you have time and use quick-cooking tools like pressure cookers or slow cookers.
- Simplified Recipes: Choose recipes with fewer ingredients and shorter preparation times.

Social Situations:

- Plan Ahead: Check the menu before eating out and decide what you'll order or suggest restaurants with healthier options.
- Bring Your Own: At social gatherings, offer to bring a dish that fits your diet, ensuring there's something suitable for you to eat.
- Cravings and Temptations:
- Healthy Alternatives: Have healthy snacks on hand to combat cravings. Nuts, seeds, and fruits are excellent choices.
- Understand Triggers: Recognize what triggers your cravings and develop strategies to address them, such as distraction, hydration, or eating balanced meals to prevent hunger spikes.

MAINTAINING MOTIVATION AND CELEBRATING MILESTONES

Long-term adherence to lifestyle changes requires sustained motivation and recognition of your achievements.

Set Clear Goals:
- SMART Goals: Ensure your goals are Specific, Measurable, Achievable, Relevant, and Time-bound.
- Small Steps: Break larger goals into smaller, manageable steps to prevent feeling overwhelmed.

Track Progress:
- Journaling: Keep a diary of your food intake, exercise, and how you feel. Reflecting on progress can provide motivation on tougher days.
- Apps and Tech: Use apps to monitor your diet, activity levels, and overall progress.

Celebrate Successes:
- Reward Yourself: Set up rewards for reaching milestones, like a new cookbook for a new diet milestone or a new outfit for weight loss goals.
- Share Your Achievements: Sharing progress with friends, family, or support groups can boost your morale and encourage continued efforts.
- Stay Flexible:
- Adapt to Changes: Be ready to adjust your goals and methods as your lifestyle, abilities, and circumstances change.
- Be Patient: Understand that progress may be slow, and setbacks are part of the journey. Persistence is key.

By navigating these challenges with determination and a flexible approach, you can maintain progress and achieve sustained success in managing your health. This journey is not just about reaching a destination but also about learning and growing along the way. Celebrate each step forward and embrace the path to better health with confidence and optimism.

GET YOUR BONUS!

Dear Valued Reader,

As you explore the recipes in our Fatty Liver Diet Cookbook, we hope you've found inspiration and guidance for preparing healthful meals that support liver health. Your decision to bring our recipes into your kitchen is greatly valued.

To show our appreciation for joining our community, we have a special gift waiting just for you. To access this token of our thanks:

Kindly scan the QR code located at the center of this page.

Be transported to an exclusive download page where your bonus content awaits—our way of saying 'Thank You'.

https://recipemaker.ck.page/fattyliver_stewartbrooks

Your enthusiasm for healthy eating fuels our commitment to continually innovate and provide you with the best recipes for a liver-friendly lifestyle. We are honored to be a part of your journey in creating nutritious and delicious meals.

Here's to many more delightful dishes and cherished moments in the kitchen.

With warmest regards,
Stewart Brooks

APPENDIX
GLOSSARY OF TERMS

Fatty Liver Disease: Also known as hepatic steatosis, this condition involves the accumulation of fat in liver cells. It can be classified as alcoholic fatty liver disease (AFLD) or non-alcoholic fatty liver disease (NAFLD), depending on the influence of alcohol consumption.

AFLD (Alcoholic Fatty Liver Disease): A condition characterized by fat accumulation in the liver as a result of excessive alcohol consumption. This can lead to liver inflammation and, eventually, more severe liver damage.

NAFLD (Non-alcoholic Fatty Liver Disease): The most common chronic liver condition, particularly in Western countries, characterized by the accumulation of fat in the liver in people who consume little or no alcohol. It is closely associated with obesity and insulin resistance.

MASLD (Metabolic Associated Steatohepatitis Liver Disease): Formerly known as NASH, this term is used to describe liver inflammation and damage caused by a build-up of fat in the liver, associated with metabolic dysfunction.

NASH (Non-alcoholic Steatohepatitis): A serious form of non-alcoholic fatty liver disease (NAFLD) characterized by liver inflammation and damage in addition to fat accumulation in the liver. This condition can lead to more severe liver damage, such as fibrosis (scarring of liver tissue), and eventually progress to cirrhosis or liver cancer if untreated. NASH often occurs in individuals who drink little or no alcohol and is commonly associated with obesity, type 2 diabetes, and metabolic syndrome. Effective management includes lifestyle changes and, as of recent developments, may include pharmacological treatments such as Rezdiffa, which has been approved by the FDA as the first specific therapy for NASH.

Rezdiffa: A pharmaceutical drug developed by Madrigal Pharmaceuticals, approved by the FDA as the first specific therapy for Non-alcoholic Steatohepatitis (NASH). Rezdiffa is designed to treat this severe form of non-alcoholic fatty liver disease, which is characterized by liver inflammation and can lead to fibrosis and cirrhosis if not managed effectively.

Zero Sugar: Foods or products that contain no sugar. These are often used in diets to control blood sugar levels or manage diabetes.

Whole Foods: Foods that are unprocessed and unrefined or processed and refined as little as possible before being consumed. Examples include whole fruits, vegetables, and grains.

Vegan: A diet and lifestyle that excludes all animal products, including meat, dairy, and eggs, often for ethical, health, or environmental reasons.

Low Glycemic: Refers to foods that do not cause large spikes in blood sugar levels based on their low ranking in the glycemic index.

Heart-Healthy: Foods or diets that contribute to the maintenance of good cardiovascular health, typically low in saturated fats, cholesterol, and sodium while rich in fiber and antioxidants.

Vegetarian: A dietary pattern that excludes meat, fish, and poultry but may include dairy products and eggs, depending on the type of vegetarian diet followed.

Gluten-Free: A diet entirely free from gluten, which is a protein found in wheat, barley, and rye, necessary for managing celiac disease or other gluten sensitivities.

Dairy-Free: A diet that excludes milk and milk products, suitable for individuals with lactose intolerance or dairy allergies or for those who avoid dairy for ethical reasons.

High-Protein: Foods or diets that are rich in protein content, important for muscle repair, immune function, and overall health maintenance.

High-Fiber: Foods or diets that have a high content of dietary fiber which aids in digestion, helps manage blood sugar levels, and reduces cholesterol.

Low Sodium: Diets that limit salt intake to reduce the risk of hypertension and cardiovascular disease.

Low-Fat: Foods or diets that contain minimal amounts of fats, particularly saturated fats and trans fats, to help maintain weight and improve heart health.

Low-Calorie: Foods or diets that provide fewer calories than standard dietary recommendations, useful for weight loss and managing caloric intake.

Vitamin A Rich: Foods high in Vitamin A, which is crucial for vision, growth, cell division, reproduction, and immunity.

Vitamin D Rich: Foods high in Vitamin D, important for the absorption of calcium, promoting bone growth, and playing a role in immune function.

Vitamin E Rich: Foods high in Vitamin E, an antioxidant that helps protect cells from the damage caused by free radicals.

Vitamin C Rich: Foods high in Vitamin C, necessary for the growth and repair of tissues in all parts of your body and are involved in many body functions, including the formation of collagen, absorption of iron, the immune system, wound healing, and the maintenance of cartilage, bones, and teeth.

RECOMMENDED APPS AND ONLINE RESOURCES

In today's digital age, managing health, particularly conditions like fatty liver disease, has been greatly facilitated by a wide array of mobile applications. These apps offer various functionalities, from tracking your daily caloric intake and physical activity to providing customized meal plans and meditation routines. With such an abundance of options available, finding the perfect app tailored to your personal health needs and preferences is more feasible than ever.

The process of selecting the right app often involves some trial and error. This journey allows you to explore different features and interfaces to determine which tools best support your lifestyle changes and health goals. Many applications offer core services at no cost, providing significant value without investment. However, for those who require more in-depth tracking, customized options, or advanced functionalities, many apps also offer additional features for a fee. It's important to assess whether these premium features justify the cost based on your specific needs.

This curated list of apps is designed to serve as a starting point in your search. It highlights key players in categories relevant to diet management, fitness tracking, and mental wellness, guiding you toward the types of apps or resources that you should consider first. Whether you are looking for a simple tool to help monitor your daily food intake or a comprehensive platform to overhaul your lifestyle, the right application can make a significant difference in effectively managing fatty liver disease and improving your overall health.

Calorie Counting Apps:

1. **FatSecret**
   - Features: Calorie counter, food diary, healthy recipes, weight tracker, and monthly summary view.
   - Advantages: Includes a community aspect for sharing and support; free to use.
   - Disadvantages: Fewer features than some competitors; limited integration with other fitness apps.
   - Price: Free.

2. **MyFitnessPal**
   - Features: Comprehensive food diary, barcode scanner, extensive food database, recipe importer, and calorie counter.
   - Advantages: Large food database; connects with various fitness trackers; provides detailed reports on nutrition and calories.
   - Disadvantages: Premium features require a subscription; some users find the app can be overwhelming due to its many features.
   - Price: Free version available; Premium at $9.99/month or $49.99/year.

3. **Lose It!**
   - Features: Allows users to set weight loss goals and track food intake using a comprehensive food database and a barcode scanner.
   - Advantages: Easy to use with a straightforward interface; provides a robust support community.
   - Disadvantages: Some users may find the free version limited, and the premium version is required for more detailed nutrient analysis.
   - Price: Free version available; Premium at $39.99/year.
4. **Cron-O-Meter**
   - Features: Offers detailed tracking of calorie intake and a breakdown of micronutrients. Users can log food, exercise, and health data.
   - Advantages: Provides precise tracking of more than 60 nutrients and syncs with several fitness apps and devices.
   - Disadvantages: The interface may not be as visually appealing as other apps; best suited for those who need detailed tracking.
   - Price: Free version available; Gold membership at $5.99/month or $39.99/year.

Product Selection and Diet Management:

1. **Yummly**
   - Features: Recipe recommendations tailored to dietary preferences and allergies, meal planning, and shopping list tools.
   - Advantages: Personalized recipe suggestions; integrates with smart kitchen devices.
   - Disadvantages: Not all recipes are vetted by nutritionists; some premium features require payment.
   - Price: Free version available; Yummly Pro is $4.99/month.
2. Fooducate
   - Features: Food grading system, calorie and exercise tracking, food diary, and diet tips.
   - Advantages: Educates users about food quality and nutrition beyond calorie counting.
   - Disadvantages: Premium features are needed for more comprehensive tracking and analysis.
   - Price: Free version available; Pro version ranges from $4.99/month to $74.99/lifetime.

3. **ShopWell**
   - Features: Barcode scanning, personalized food recommendations based on health goals and dietary needs.
   - Advantages: Helps users find foods that match their dietary requirements, such as low sodium or high fiber, which is crucial for managing fatty liver.
   - Disadvantages: The database is not as extensive as some other apps, which might limit food discovery.
   - Price: Free

4. **Fig**
   - Features: Food label transparency tool that helps users understand the nutritional content and ingredients of food products.
   - Advantages: Offers detailed breakdowns of food labels, making it easier for users to avoid specific ingredients for health reasons.
   - Disadvantages: New app with a growing database, so some products might not yet be included.
   - Price: Free.

5. **Eat This Much**
   - Features: Automatic meal planner that generates daily meal plans based on calorie goals and food preferences.
   - Advantages: Ideal for strict diet adherence, providing precise meal planning and grocery lists.
   - Disadvantages: Full functionality requires a subscription; some users might find the meal plans too rigid.
   - Price: Free version available; Premium at $8.99/month.

Fitness Apps:

1. **Strava**
   - Features: Tracks cycling, running, and swimming with GPS; includes social features to connect with friends and participate in challenges.
   - Advantages: Great for outdoor activities with a strong community aspect; motivating for those who enjoy competition.
   - Disadvantages: Some advanced features, such as detailed analytics and personalized coaching, require a subscription.
   - Price: Free version available; Premium (Strava Summit) at $5.00/month.

2. **Fitbit App**
   - Features: Activity tracking, sleep monitoring, heart rate monitoring, food logging.
   - Advantages: Comprehensive health tracking when used with a Fitbit device motivational challenges.
   - Disadvantages: Limited use without a Fitbit device; some features locked behind a subscription.
   - Price: Free basic app; Fitbit Premium at $9.99/month or $79.99/year.

3. **7 Minute Workout**
   - Features: Quick, high-intensity workouts that can be done at home with no equipment.
   - Advantages: Ideal for busy individuals; scientifically proven to improve fitness.
   - Disadvantages: Might be too basic for more advanced fitness enthusiasts.
   - Price: Free; offers in-app purchases.

4. **Daily Burn**
   - Features: Provides a variety of daily workout videos tailored to your fitness goals, including beginner-friendly routines.
   - Advantages: Extensive library of workouts; live classes available daily.
   - Disadvantages: Requires a subscription for all features and content.
   - Price: Starts at $14.95/month after a 30-day free trial.

Meditation Apps:

1. **Calm**
   - Features: Guided meditations, sleep stories, breathing exercises, and relaxing music.
   - Advantages: Wide variety of content aimed at reducing stress and improving sleep quality.
   - Disadvantages: Premium content can be costly.
   - Price: Free limited version; Premium at $69.99/year.

2. **10% Happier**
   - Features: Guided meditations, videos, and sleep content designed with a practical, no-nonsense approach to mindfulness.
   - Advantages: Features well-known meditation teachers; focuses on practical mindfulness skills.
   - Disadvantages: Requires a subscription for full access to all features.
   - Price: Free limited version; Premium at $99/year.

3. **Breethe**
- Features: Guided meditations, life coaching, masterclasses, music, and bedtime stories.
- Advantages: Holistic approach covering various aspects of mental wellness including relationships and personal growth.
- Disadvantages: Premium subscription is needed for complete access.
- Price: $12.95/month or $89.95/year after a free trial.

Apps for Emotional Support:

1. **Woebot**
- Features: An AI-powered chatbot that provides emotional support through therapeutic conversations and CBT techniques.
- Advantages: Accessible and user-friendly; good for daily mental health check-ins.
- Disadvantages: AI may not fully replace the nuanced understanding of a human therapist.
- Price: Free.

2. **Sanvello**
- Features: On-demand help with stress, anxiety, and depression through cognitive behavioral therapy (CBT) techniques, guided meditations, and progress tracking.
- Advantages: Offers tools based on clinically validated techniques; free access to peer support community.
- Disadvantages: Some features are only available with Premium.
- Price: Free basic version; Premium at $8.99/month.

3. **BetterHelp**
- Features: Online counseling and therapy services with licensed therapists.
- Advantages: Wide range of counseling specialties available; flexible communication methods.
- Disadvantages: Cost may be a barrier for some; not covered by insurance.
- Price: Typically ranges from $60 to $90 per week, billed monthly.

INDEX

A

Air-Fried Spiced Carrot Chips 72

Almond Butter and Banana Oatmeal 39

Asian-Style Turkey Meatballs with Vegetable Stir Fry 89

Asparagus and Shrimp with Quinoa 52

Avocado and Lime Frozen Yogurt 79

Avocado Cocoa Mousse 103

B

Baked Cod Fish Sticks with Yogurt Dill Sauce 75

Baked Grapefruit with Cinnamon 103

Baked Hake with Sweet Potato Wedges 63

Baked Peaches with Crushed Almonds 108

Balsamic Glazed Duck Breast with Pear Chutney 90

Balsamic Grilled Zucchini with Parmesan 52

Beef and Vegetable Kebabs with Tzatziki 91

Beetroot and Carrot Juice Cleanse 41

Black Bean and Butternut Squash Stew 81

Blackened Catfish with Collard Greens 60

Blueberry and Lemon Chia Fresca 105

Broccoli and Feta Cheese Scramble 42

Butternut Squash and Chickpea Curry 51

Butternut Squash and Sage Risotto 63

C

Carrot and Ginger Purée Soup 47

Carrot, Orange, and Ginger Immune Booster 112

Chia Seed and Raspberry Pudding 43

Chilled Mango Soup with Mint 106

Citrus Roasted Turkey Breast 59

Coconut and Lime Rice Pudding 108

Cod and Parsnip Stew 81

Cod in Parsley Cream Sauce 61

Cottage Cheese Pancakes with Blueberries 34

Creamy Avocado and Cucumber Soup 86

Creamy Broccoli and Spinach Soup 56

Cucumber Boats with Spicy Shrimp Salad 73

Cucumber, Celery, and Lime Hydration Drink 112

D

Date and Nut Truffles 107

E

Eggplant Rollatini with Spinach and Ricotta 53

F

Fresh Berry Salad with Mint 107

G

Garlic Roasted Trout with Brussels Sprouts 49

Green Tea Infusion with Mint and Lemon 113

Green Tea Yogurt Parfait 42

Grilled Chicken and Avocado Wrap 39

Grilled Haddock with Olive Tapenade 46

Grilled Halibut with Citrus Salsa 66

Grilled Swordfish with Mediterranean Salad 62

Grilled Tuna with a Citrus Tomato Salsa 100

H

Hearty Minestrone Soup with Whole Wheat Pasta 46

Herb Roasted Chicken with Root Vegetables 68

Horseradish Encrusted Salmon with Beetroot Salad 96

K

Kale and Apple Chips 76

Kale and White Bean Soup 85

L

Lemon and Dill Poached Salmon 99

Lemon and Herb Poached Haddock 70

Lemon Garlic Tilapia with Steamed Kale 53

Lemon-Pepper Cod with Broccoli Puree 97

M

Mango and Coconut Chia Pudding 41

Mango, Kiwi, and Spinach Smoothie 115

Maple-Glazed Arctic Char with Braised Leeks 97

Matcha and Spirulina Energy Drink 114

Minty Pea and Avocado Spread on Whole Grain Toast 78

Miso Glazed Black Cod with Stir-Fried Greens 100

Miso-Glazed Cod with Bok Choy 67

Mixed Berry Whole Grain Porridge 40

Moroccan Spiced Chicken Stew with Apricots 88

Moroccan Spiced Fish with Couscous 65

Mushroom and Barley Soup 83

N

No-Bake Walnut and Date Energy Balls 79

P

Parchment-Baked Halibut with Asparagus 95

Pear and Ginger Compote 104

Pear and Ginger Soother 117

Pear and Walnut Oatmeal 35

Pesto Chicken and Veggie Wrap 54

Pineapple and Fresh Turmeric Digestive Aid 114

Pineapple Carpaccio with Fresh Basil 102

Pumpkin and Black Bean Casserole 56

Pumpkin and Chickpea Stew 82

Pumpkin Curry with Brown Rice 69

Pumpkin Hummus with Whole Grain Pita Chips 76

Pumpkin Spice Energy Balls 102

Q

Quinoa and Apple Breakfast Bowl 38

Quinoa Tabbouleh with Chickpeas 45

R

Raspberry Coconut Chia Pudding 106

Raspberry, Lime, and Coconut Water Slushie 113

Ricotta and Berry Stuffed Celery 74

Roasted Beet and Feta Salad 61

Roasted Brussels Sprouts and Pomegranate Salad 67

Roasted Brussels Sprouts with Lemon Dip 73

Roasted Cauliflower and Chickpea Tacos 59

Roasted Cinnamon Hazelnuts 59

Roasted Turmeric and Cumin Cauliflower Bites 78

Roasted Vegetable and Farro Bowl 50

S

Salmon and Avocado Toast 38

Sautéed Brussels Sprouts with Crispy Tofu 57

Seared Scallops with Quinoa and Apple Salad 68

Slow-Cooked Turkey Chili with Sweet Potatoes 90

Smoked Salmon and Avocado Toast 34

Smoked Salmon and Cream Cheese Cucumber Rolls 72

Soothing Chamomile and Lavender Tea 115

Soy-Ginger Glazed Salmon with Bok Choy 95

Spaghetti Squash and Meatballs with Tomato Basil Sauce 93

Spaghetti Squash Pad Thai 65

Spiced Chicken Skewers with Yogurt Cucumber Dip 92

Spiced Lentil Stew with Coconut Milk 47

Spiced Monkfish with Lentil Dal 98

Spiced Pumpkin Porridge 36

Spicy Tofu and Bok Choy Stir-Fry 66

Spicy Tomato and Lentil Soup 85

Spinach and Egg White Omelette 40

Spinach and Mushroom Polenta Stacks 50

Steamed Mussels with Garlic and Herbs 99

Stir-Fried Beef and Broccoli with Tamari Sauce 92

Stir-Fried Kale and Quinoa 60

Stuffed Cherry Tomatoes with Tuna Salad 77

Stuffed Peppers with Ground Chicken and Brown Rice 89

Stuffed Portobello Mushrooms with Spinach and Pine Nuts 57

Sugar-Free Almond Butter Brownies 110

T

Tahini and Cocoa Energy Bites 77

Tuna and White Bean Salad 48

Turkey and Quinoa Stew 83

Turmeric and Pineapple Anti-Inflammatory Smoothie 57

Turmeric Grilled Chicken and Quinoa Salad 110

V

Vegan Buddha Bowl with Spiced Chickpeas 49

Vegan Mushroom and Lentil Bolognese 70

Vegan Tofu Scramble with Spinach and Tomatoes 35

Vegetable and Tempeh Stew 84

Vegetable and Tofu Pad Thai 58

Vegetable Hash with Poached Egg 37

W

Walnut and Pear Oat Bake 37

Whole Wheat Pancakes with Fresh Fruit 43

Z

Zucchini and Chocolate Chip Bread (Sugar-Free) 109

Zucchini and Herb Fritters 74

Made in United States
Orlando, FL
20 June 2024